Drug Speller
2012

ISBN-10: 1467926604
EAN-13: 9781467926607
Library of Congress Control Number:

Drug Speller 2012

Dictionary Jumpstart, Inc.

Drug Speller 2012

Dictionary Jumpstart

NOTICE

Many of the drugs and/or products listed in this publication are protected by copyright, trademark or patent law and such designations are omitted for ease of use in this publication.

TYPOGRAPHY

Various drug and medical product manufacturers prefer specific typographical characterizations of their products such as the mixing of upper and lower case letters and the insertion of hyphens, et cetera… Where possible, these preferences have been followed. However, these proprietary preferences are often disregarded in medical literature. Therefore, this book has chosen to use the most common typographical representations of drugs and/or products.

While every effort has been made to assure the accuracy of the spellings and categorizations contained in this publication, errors can occur and the author is not liable for any damages arising from the use or misuse of this publication. Furthermore, drugs are commonly used in multiple medical specialities for diverse reasons. The author's categorization of drugs is based upon the more common use of the drugs so categorized.

RECOMMENDED USE OF THIS BOOK

This publication is designed to be used only by skilled professionals in researching the spelling of terminology. It should not be used for the prescribing or the taking of medication or in determining the proper use of drugs and/or medical products.

This publication is divided into two parts. The first part is an alphabetical listing of drugs; prescription, over the counter, brand name, generic name, discontinued, new approvals and experimental. The second half is broken down as indicated in the Index on the cover of the book by medical category. The two parts are divided by the "Categorically" page.

Nothing in this book should be construed as endorsing or recommending any drug or medical product.

Due to publishing deadlines, this book is up to date through October 31, 2011.

Copies of this book can be purchased online at **www.drugspeller.com**

A

- 13-Valent Vaccine
- 4-aminopyridine
- A+D
- abacavir
- abatacept
- Abbokinase
- Abbo-Pac
- abciximab
- Abelcet
- Abilify
- Abilify Discmelt
- Abiraterone
- abobotulinumtoxinA
- Abraxane
- Abreva
- Absorbine Jr.
- Abstral
- ABthrax
- ABX-EGF
- AC2993
- ACAM2000
- ACZ885
- acamprosate
- Acanya
- acarbose
- Accolate
- Accretropin
- Accuflora
- AccuNeb
- Accupril
- Accurbron
- Accuretic
- Accutane
- Accuzyme
- acebutolol
- ACE inhibitors
- Acel-Imune
- Aceon

A

- Acephen
- ACES
- Acetadote
- acetaminophen
- Acetasol
- Acetavance
- acetazolamide
- acetohexamide
- acetohydroxamic acid
- acetyl sulfisoxazole
- acetylcysteine
- acetylsalicylic acid
- Achromycin
- acid mantle creme
- acid phosphatase
- Aci-Jel
- AcipHex
- acitretin
- Aclasta
- aclidinium bromide
- Aclovate
- AcneFree
- Acomplia
- Acova
- Acrivastine
- Actemra
- ACTH
- Acthar
- Acthar Gel
- Acthrel
- ActHIB
- Actical
- Acticin
- Actidel
- Actidose
- Actidose-Aqua
- Actifade
- Actifed

A

- ❑ Actigall
- ❑ Actimmune
- ❑ Actin
- ❑ Actiq
- ❑ ACTIS
- ❑ Activase
- ❑ Activella
- ❑ Activelle
- ❑ Activ On
- ❑ Actiza
- ❑ Actonel
- ❑ ACTOplus met
- ❑ Actos
- ❑ Acular
- ❑ Acuprin 81
- ❑ Acurox
- ❑ Acutrim
- ❑ Acuvail
- ❑ acyclovir
- ❑ acycloguanosine
- ❑ Aczone
- ❑ Adacel
- ❑ Adagen
- ❑ Adalat
- ❑ Adalimumab
- ❑ Adamet
- ❑ adapalene
- ❑ Adasuve
- ❑ Adcetris
- ❑ Adcirca
- ❑ Adderall
- ❑ Adeflor M
- ❑ Adefovir dipivoxil
- ❑ Adenocard
- ❑ Adenoscan
- ❑ adenosine
- ❑ Adipex
- ❑ Adipex-P

A

- ❑ Adoxa
- ❑ adrenocorticoids
- ❑ Adriamycin
- ❑ Adriana
- ❑ Adrucil
- ❑ Adsorbocarpine
- ❑ Advair Diskus
- ❑ Advair HFA
- ❑ Advate
- ❑ Advicor
- ❑ Advil
- ❑ Advil Liqui-Gels
- ❑ AeroBid
- ❑ AeroChamber
- ❑ AeroCount
- ❑ Aerolate
- ❑ Aerolone
- ❑ Aerophylline
- ❑ Aeroseb-DX
- ❑ Aerosporin
- ❑ Afeditab CR
- ❑ Affinitak
- ❑ Afinitor
- ❑ Aflaxen
- ❑ Aflexa
- ❑ aflibercept
- ❑ Aftate
- ❑ Afluria
- ❑ Afresa
- ❑ Afrezza
- ❑ Afrin
- ❑ Aftate
- ❑ Agalsidase
- ❑ Agenerase
- ❑ aggrastat
- ❑ Aggrenox
- ❑ Agoral
- ❑ Agriflu

A

- ❏ Agrylin
- ❏ AHA
- ❏ AH-Chew
- ❏ AHF
- ❏ A-Hydrocort
- ❏ AidsVax
- ❏ Airet
- ❏ AK-Chlor
- ❏ AK-Con
- ❏ AK-Dilate
- ❏ AK-Fluor
- ❏ Akineton
- ❏ Akne-Mycin
- ❏ AK-Nefrin
- ❏ Akorn antioxidants
- ❏ AK-Pentolate
- ❏ AK-Poly
- ❏ AK-Pred
- ❏ Akpro
- ❏ Akrinol
- ❏ AK-Rinse
- ❏ AK-Spore
- ❏ AK-Sulf
- ❏ Akten
- ❏ Aktob
- ❏ AK-Tracin
- ❏ AK-Trol
- ❏ Akwa Tears
- ❏ ALA
- ❏ Alacol DM Syrup
- ❏ Alamast
- ❏ alatrofloxacin
- ❏ Alavert
- ❏ Alaway
- ❏ Alba
- ❏ Albalon
- ❏ Albamycin
- ❏ Albatussin SR

A

- ❏ albendazole
- ❏ Albenza
- ❏ albinterferon alfa-2b
- ❏ Albolene
- ❏ albuferon
- ❏ Albumarc
- ❏ albumin
- ❏ Albuminar
- ❏ Albutein
- ❏ albuterol
- ❏ albuterol sulfate
- ❏ alcaftadine
- ❏ Alcaine
- ❏ alclometasone
- ❏ Alcomicin
- ❏ Alconefrin 12
- ❏ Aldactazide
- ❏ Aldactone
- ❏ Aldara
- ❏ aldesleukin
- ❏ Aldoclor
- ❏ Aldomet
- ❏ Aldoril
- ❏ Aldurazyme
- ❏ Alefacept
- ❏ Alemtuzumab
- ❏ alendronate
- ❏ Aleve
- ❏ Aleve-D
- ❏ Alfenta
- ❏ Alfentanil
- ❏ Alferon N
- ❏ alfuzosin
- ❏ algalsidase alfa
- ❏ agalsidase beta
- ❏ Alglucerase
- ❏ alglucosidase alfa
- ❏ Align

A

- Alimentum Protein
- Alimta
- Alinia
- aliskiren
- AlitraQ Nutrition
- Alitretinoin
- alkaline phosphatase
- Alka-Mints
- Alka-Seltzer
- Alka-Seltzer Plus
- Alkeran
- Allantoin
- All-Basic
- Allegra
- Allegra-D
- AllerNaze
- AlleRx
- Allfen
- Alli
- allium cepa
- allobarbital
- allopurinol
- almotriptan
- almotriptan malate
- Alocril
- aloe vera
- alogliptin
- Alomide
- Alophen
- Aloprim
- Alora
- alosetron
- Aloxi
- alpha1-proteinase
- alpha adrenergic receptor blockers
- alpha chymotrypsin
- alpha-galactosidase
- Alphagan

A

- Alpha-Hydroxy
- Alpha Keri
- alpha-linolenic acid
- Alpha Lipoic
- Alphanate
- AlphaNine
- alpha-proteinase
- Alpha Tocopherol
- Alphatrex
- alprazolam
- alprostadil
- Alrex
- Alsuma
- Altabax
- Altace
- alteplase
- Alternagel
- Altinac
- Altocor
- Altoprev
- Altramucil
- altretamine
- Alu-Cap
- Aludrox
- Alumadrine
- aluminum acetate
- aluminum hydroxide
- Alupent
- Alustra
- Alvesco
- alvimopan
- amantadine
- Amaryl
- Ambenyl
- Ambi
- Ambien
- Ambifed
- AmBisome

A

- ambrisentan
- amcinonide
- Amdoxovir
- Amen
- Amerge
- Americaine
- Amerifed
- Amerituss AD
- Amertan
- AmethaPred
- Amethopterin
- Amevive
- Amfedsul
- AMG 073
- Amicar
- Amidate
- amifostine
- Amigen
- Amikacin
- Amikin
- amiloride
- amino acid
- Amino-cerv
- aminobenzoate
- aminocaproic acid
- aminoglutethimide
- aminoglycoside
- aminohippurate
- Aminolete
- aminolevulinic acid
- Aminomine
- aminophylline
- Aminoplex
- aminosalicylic acid
- Aminostasis
- Aminosyn
- Aminotate
- Aminovirox

A

- Aminoxin
- amiodarone
- amithiozone
- Amitiza
- Amitone
- amitriptyline
- AmLactin AP
- AmLactin XL
- amlexanox
- amlodipine
- amlodipine besylate
- ammonium chloride
- ammonium lactate
- Ammonul
- Amnesteem
- Amnestrogen
- amobarbital
- Amox Clav Pot
- amoxapine
- amoxicillin
- Amoxil
- ampakine
- Amphadase
- Amphedroxyn
- amphetamine
- Amphojel
- Amphotec
- amphotericin
- Ampicin
- ampicillin
- Ampligen
- amprenavir
- Ampyra
- amrinone lactate
- Amrix
- Amsustain
- Amturnide
- Amvaz

A

- ❑ Amylase
- ❑ amyl nitrate
- ❑ Amytal Sodium
- ❑ Amyvid
- ❑ Anabar
- ❑ Anacel
- ❑ Anacin
- ❑ Anadrol
- ❑ Anafranil
- ❑ anagrelide
- ❑ Anakinra
- ❑ Ana-Kit
- ❑ Analpram
- ❑ ananas comosus
- ❑ Anaplex
- ❑ Anaprox
- ❑ Anascorp
- ❑ Anaspaz
- ❑ anastrozole
- ❑ Anatrast
- ❑ Anatuss
- ❑ Anbesol
- ❑ Ancef
- ❑ Ancobon
- ❑ Ancrod
- ❑ Androderm
- ❑ AndroGel
- ❑ Android
- ❑ Andropository injection
- ❑ Andro-Teston
- ❑ Androxal
- ❑ AN-DTPA Kit
- ❑ Anectine
- ❑ Anestacon
- ❑ Anesthesin
- ❑ Anexsia
- ❑ Angeliq
- ❑ Angio Conray

A

- ❑ Angiomax
- ❑ Angiovist
- ❑ Anhydron
- ❑ anidulafungin
- ❑ aniledrine
- ❑ Animi-3
- ❑ Anisindione
- ❑ anistreplase
- ❑ Anolor
- ❑ Ansaid
- ❑ Ansamycin
- ❑ Antabuse
- ❑ antacids
- ❑ Antagon
- ❑ Antara
- ❑ Antegren
- ❑ anthelmintics
- ❑ anthracycline
- ❑ anthralin
- ❑ AntiBetic
- ❑ Antibiopto
- ❑ antihemophilic factor
- ❑ antihistamines
- ❑ Anti-Ige
- ❑ Anti-Inhibitor
- ❑ Antilirium
- ❑ antipyrine
- ❑ antithrombin
- ❑ anti-thymocyte globulin
- ❑ ANTIOX
- ❑ antipyrine
- ❑ Antivenin
- ❑ Antivert
- ❑ Antizol
- ❑ Antrocol
- ❑ Anturane
- ❑ Anturol
- ❑ Anusol

A

- ❑ ANX-530
- ❑ Anzemet
- ❑ Ao-Zidovudine
- ❑ APAP elixir
- ❑ Apatate
- ❑ APC
- ❑ APC8015
- ❑ Apcitide
- ❑ APF530
- ❑ Aphrodyne
- ❑ Aphthasol
- ❑ A.P.I.
- ❑ Apidra
- ❑ APL
- ❑ Aplenzin
- ❑ Aplisol
- ❑ ApoA-1
- ❑ ApoA-1 Milano
- ❑ Apokyn
- ❑ apomorphine hydrochloride
- ❑ Appearex
- ❑ apraclonidine
- ❑ aprepitant
- ❑ Apriso
- ❑ Apresazide
- ❑ Apresoline
- ❑ Apri
- ❑ aprobarbital
- ❑ aprotinin
- ❑ APSAC
- ❑ Aptivus
- ❑ Aqua-Ban
- ❑ Aquachloral
- ❑ AquaLase
- ❑ AquaMEPHYTON
- ❑ Aquanil
- ❑ Aquaphor
- ❑ Aquaphyllin

A

- ❑ Aquasol
- ❑ Aquatar
- ❑ Aquatensen
- ❑ Aquavan
- ❑ Aquify
- ❑ Ara-C
- ❑ Aralast NP
- ❑ Aralen
- ❑ Aramine
- ❑ Aranesp
- ❑ Arava
- ❑ Arbutamine
- ❑ Arcalyst
- ❑ Arcapta
- ❑ Arco-Lase
- ❑ Ardeparin
- ❑ Arduan
- ❑ Aredia
- ❑ Arestin
- ❑ Arfonad
- ❑ arformoterol tartrate
- ❑ argatroban
- ❑ ArginMax
- ❑ Aricept
- ❑ Aridol
- ❑ Arimidex
- ❑ aripiprazole
- ❑ Aristocort
- ❑ AristoDerm
- ❑ Aristospan
- ❑ Arixtra
- ❑ Arm-A-Med
- ❑ armodafinil
- ❑ Aromasin
- ❑ Arranon
- ❑ arsenic trioxide
- ❑ Artane
- ❑ Artecoll

A

- Artefill
- artemether
- Arth Arrest
- Arth DR
- ArthriCare
- ArthriFlex
- Arthriten
- Arthritis-Patch
- Arthro-7
- Arthrotec
- Arth-Rx
- Arthur It is
- Artiss
- Arzerra
- Aryplase
- Asacol
- Asbron
- Ascensia Breeze
- Asclera
- ascorbic acid
- Ascriptin
- asenapine
- Asendin
- Asimia
- Asmalix
- Asmanex Twisthaler
- asparaginase
- Aspercreme
- Aspergum
- aspirin
- Astelin
- astemizole
- Astepro
- Asthmahaler
- Astragalus
- Astramorph
- Astring-O-Sol
- Atabrine

A

- Atacand
- Atamet
- Atapryl
- Atarax
- atazanavir
- Atelvia
- atenolol
- Atgam
- Ativan
- ATNAA
- ATnativ
- atomoxetine HCI
- Atopiclair
- atorvastatin
- atovaquone
- ATP
- atracurium
- Atrac-Tain
- Atralin
- Atretol
- Atridox
- Atripla
- Atrohist
- Atromid-S
- AtroPen
- Atropine
- Atrosept
- Atrovent
- ATryn
- A/T/S
- Attapulgite
- Attenuvax
- Aubagio
- Augmentin
- Augmentin XR
- Auralgan
- auranofin
- Aureomycin

A

- ❑ aurothioglucose
- ❑ Auroto Otic
- ❑ Australian Gold
- ❑ Auszyme
- ❑ Authia
- ❑ Autoplex
- ❑ Avagard
- ❑ Avage
- ❑ Avalide
- ❑ Avalon Organics
- ❑ Avanafil
- ❑ Avandamet
- ❑ Avandaryl
- ❑ Avandia
- ❑ Avapro
- ❑ Avastin
- ❑ AVC
- ❑ Aveed
- ❑ Aveeno
- ❑ Aveenobar
- ❑ Avelox
- ❑ Aventyl
- ❑ Aviane
- ❑ Avimil
- ❑ Avinza
- ❑ Avirax
- ❑ Avita
- ❑ Avlimil
- ❑ Avlosulfon
- ❑ Avobenzone
- ❑ Avodart
- ❑ Avonex
- ❑ AVX101
- ❑ Axert
- ❑ Axid
- ❑ Axiron
- ❑ axitinib
- ❑ Axokine
- ❑ Axotal

A

- ❑ Aygestin
- ❑ Ayr saline mist
- ❑ AZ-004
- ❑ azacitidine
- ❑ Azactam
- ❑ azafluoroquinolone
- ❑ Azasan
- ❑ AzaSite
- ❑ azatadine
- ❑ Azathioprine
- ❑ Azdone
- ❑ azelaic acid
- ❑ azelastine
- ❑ Azelex
- ❑ Azfibrocel-T
- ❑ azficel-T
- ❑ azidothymidine
- ❑ Azilect
- ❑ azilsartan medoxomil
- ❑ azithromycin
- ❑ Azmacort
- ❑ Azo
- ❑ Azo Gantanol
- ❑ Azo Gantrisin
- ❑ Azo-Standard
- ❑ Azopt
- ❑ Azor
- ❑ AZT
- ❑ aztreonam
- ❑ aztreonam lysine
- ❑ Azulfidine

B

- ❑ Babylax
- ❑ bacampicillin
- ❑ Baciquent
- ❑ bacitracin
- ❑ Bacitraycin

B	**B**

- ❑ Backaid
- ❑ baclofen
- ❑ Bacotracom
- ❑ Bactine
- ❑ Bactocill
- ❑ Bactome
- ❑ Bactrim
- ❑ Bactroban
- ❑ Bain de Soleil
- ❑ Balagan
- ❑ Balamine
- ❑ Baldex
- ❑ BAL in oil
- ❑ Balmex
- ❑ balsalazide
- ❑ balsam Peru
- ❑ Baltussin
- ❑ Banan
- ❑ Banana Boat
- ❑ Bancap HC
- ❑ Band-Aid Scar
- ❑ Banflex
- ❑ Banthine
- ❑ Banzel
- ❑ Baraclude
- ❑ Barbasol
- ❑ barbital
- ❑ barbiturates
- ❑ Baricon
- ❑ Baridol
- ❑ barium sulfate
- ❑ Barobag
- ❑ Baro-CAT
- ❑ Baroflave
- ❑ Barosperse
- ❑ Barotrast
- ❑ Bar-test
- ❑ Basaljel

- ❑ basiliximab
- ❑ Baycol
- ❑ Bayer aspirin
- ❑ BayGam
- ❑ BayHep
- ❑ BayRab
- ❑ BayRho
- ❑ BayTet
- ❑ BCG vaccine
- ❑ BCNU
- ❑ BDP Nasal
- ❑ Beano
- ❑ Beano Meltaways
- ❑ Bebulin
- ❑ becaplermin
- ❑ beclomethasone
- ❑ Beclovent
- ❑ Beconase
- ❑ Beelith
- ❑ Beepen
- ❑ belatacept
- ❑ belimumab
- ❑ belladonna alkaloids
- ❑ Bellatal
- ❑ Bellergal
- ❑ Belotero Balance
- ❑ benactyzine
- ❑ Benadryl
- ❑ Benadryl-D
- ❑ benazepril
- ❑ bendamustine
- ❑ bendroflumethiazide
- ❑ Benefiber
- ❑ BeneFix
- ❑ BeneJoint
- ❑ Benemid
- ❑ BENGAY
- ❑ Benicar

B	B

- ❑ Benlysta
- ❑ Benoquin
- ❑ Benoxinate
- ❑ Bensulfoid
- ❑ bentoquatam
- ❑ Bentyl
- ❑ Benylin
- ❑ Benzac
- ❑ BenzaClin gel
- ❑ Benzagel
- ❑ benzalkonium
- ❑ Benzamycin
- ❑ Benzashave
- ❑ Benzedrex
- ❑ Benzedrine
- ❑ benzethonium
- ❑ Benziq
- ❑ benzocaine
- ❑ Benzodent
- ❑ benzodiazepine
- ❑ benzoic acid
- ❑ benzonatate
- ❑ benzoyl peroxide
- ❑ benzphetamine
- ❑ benzquinamide
- ❑ benzthiazide
- ❑ benztropine mesylate
- ❑ benzydamine
- ❑ benzyl alcohol
- ❑ Bepadin
- ❑ bepotastine
- ❑ Bepreve
- ❑ bepridil
- ❑ beractant
- ❑ Berinert
- ❑ besifloxacin
- ❑ Besivance
- ❑ BeStent

- ❑ BeSure
- ❑ beta-adrenergic blockers
- ❑ beta carotene
- ❑ beta lactamase
- ❑ Betadine
- ❑ Betagan
- ❑ Betaine
- ❑ beta-lactam
- ❑ Betaloc
- ❑ betamethasone
- ❑ betamethasone dipropionate
- ❑ betamethasone valerate
- ❑ Betapace
- ❑ Betasept
- ❑ Betaseron
- ❑ Betatrex
- ❑ betaxolol
- ❑ Betaxon
- ❑ bethanechol
- ❑ Betimol
- ❑ Betoptic
- ❑ bevacizumab
- ❑ Bevitamel
- ❑ bexarotene
- ❑ Bextra
- ❑ Bexxar
- ❑ Beyaz
- ❑ Biavax
- ❑ Biaxin
- ❑ bicalutamide
- ❑ bicarbonate of soda
- ❑ bichloracetic acid
- ❑ Bicillin
- ❑ Bicitra
- ❑ BiCNU
- ❑ BiCozene Cream
- ❑ BiDil
- ❑ bifidobacteria

B

- ❏ Bijuva
- ❏ Bilagog
- ❏ Bilopaque
- ❏ Biltricide
- ❏ bimatoprost
- ❏ binodenoson
- ❏ Biocef
- ❏ Bioclate
- ❏ Bio-E-Gel
- ❏ Bio Ginkgo
- ❏ BioGlue
- ❏ Biohist
- ❏ BioLean
- ❏ BioLon
- ❏ BioMD Nutraceuticals
- ❏ Bion Tears
- ❏ Biore
- ❏ Boiron
- ❏ Bio St. John's wort
- ❏ Biotin
- ❏ Bio-Tab
- ❏ Biotest Hot-Rox
- ❏ BioThrax
- ❏ Biotin
- ❏ Biozole
- ❏ biperiden
- ❏ biphetamine
- ❏ bisacodyl
- ❏ biskalcitrate
- ❏ bismuth subsalicylate
- ❏ bisoprolol
- ❏ bitolterol mesylate
- ❏ bivalirudin
- ❏ Black Cohash
- ❏ BleedArrest
- ❏ Blenoxane
- ❏ bleomycin

B

- ❏ Bleph-10
- ❏ Blephamide
- ❏ Blink
- ❏ Blinx
- ❏ Blistex
- ❏ Blocadren
- ❏ B-Long
- ❏ Bluboro
- ❏ Blu-Emu
- ❏ B & O Supprettes
- ❏ boceprevir
- ❏ Bonamil
- ❏ Bonine
- ❏ Boniva
- ❏ Bontril PDM
- ❏ Boostrix
- ❏ Borofax
- ❏ Boroleum
- ❏ bortezomib
- ❏ bosentan
- ❏ Botox
- ❏ botulinum toxin type
- ❏ BranchAmin
- ❏ Bravelle
- ❏ Breathe Right
- ❏ BreathTek UBT
- ❏ Breeze2
- ❏ Brentuximab vedotin
- ❏ Breonesin
- ❏ Brethaire
- ❏ Brethine
- ❏ Bretylate
- ❏ bretylium tosylate
- ❏ Brevibloc
- ❏ Brevicon
- ❏ Brevital, sodium
- ❏ Brevoxyl

B

- ❑ Brexin
- ❑ briazolamide
- ❑ Bricanyl
- ❑ Brilinta
- ❑ brimonidine
- ❑ brinzolamide
- ❑ Brioschi Powder
- ❑ Bromarest DX
- ❑ Bromday
- ❑ bromelain
- ❑ Bromfed
- ❑ bromfenac
- ❑ bromocriptine
- ❑ bromocriptine mesylate
- ❑ bromonidine
- ❑ Bromo Quinine
- ❑ brompheniramine
- ❑ Bromural
- ❑ bronchodilators, adrenergic
- ❑ bronchodilators, xanthine
- ❑ Broncholate
- ❑ Bronkaid
- ❑ Bronkodyl
- ❑ Bronkometer aerosol
- ❑ Bronkosol
- ❑ Brontex
- ❑ Brovana
- ❑ brucine poison
- ❑ Bryostatin
- ❑ BSS
- ❑ bucindolol
- ❑ buclizine
- ❑ budesonide
- ❑ bufexamac
- ❑ BufferGel
- ❑ Bufferin
- ❑ Bufopto
- ❑ Bull Frog

B

- ❑ Bumetanide
- ❑ Bumex
- ❑ Buminate
- ❑ Bupap
- ❑ bupivacaine
- ❑ Buprenex
- ❑ buprenorphine
- ❑ bupropion
- ❑ Burn-A-Lay
- ❑ Burnicin
- ❑ Burn-Quel
- ❑ Buro-Sol
- ❑ Burow's solution
- ❑ Burt's Bees
- ❑ Buserelin
- ❑ BuSpar
- ❑ buspirone
- ❑ busulfan
- ❑ busulfex
- ❑ butabarbital
- ❑ butalbital
- ❑ butaperazine
- ❑ Butazolidin
- ❑ butenafine
- ❑ Butesin
- ❑ buthiazide
- ❑ Butisol
- ❑ butoconazole
- ❑ butorphanol
- ❑ Butrans
- ❑ butriptyline
- ❑ butyl aminobenzoate
- ❑ butylparaben
- ❑ butynamine
- ❑ butyrophenone
- ❑ Bydureon
- ❑ Byetta
- ❑ Bystolic

C

- ❑ C1-esterase inhibitor
- ❑ C1 inhibitor
- ❑ cabergoline
- ❑ cactinomycin
- ❑ Caduet
- ❑ CAE-SCAN
- ❑ Cafcit
- ❑ Cafergot
- ❑ caffeine
- ❑ Caladryl
- ❑ CalaGel
- ❑ Calahist
- ❑ Calamatum
- ❑ Calamine
- ❑ Calan
- ❑ Calcet
- ❑ Calcibind
- ❑ Calci-Chew
- ❑ calcifediol
- ❑ Calciferol
- ❑ Calcijex
- ❑ Calcimar
- ❑ Calci-Mix
- ❑ calcipotriene
- ❑ calcitonin
- ❑ Calcitonin-Salmon
- ❑ calcitriol
- ❑ calcium
- ❑ calcium acetate
- ❑ calcium carbonate
- ❑ calcium channel blockers
- ❑ calcium chloride
- ❑ calcium citrate
- ❑ calcium disodium
- ❑ calcium gluceptate
- ❑ calcium gluconate
- ❑ Calderol
- ❑ Caldesene

C

- ❑ Caldolor
- ❑ Calel-D
- ❑ calfactant
- ❑ Calm Colon
- ❑ CaloMist
- ❑ Calphosan
- ❑ Caltrate
- ❑ calvacin
- ❑ Cama Arthritis
- ❑ Camalox
- ❑ Cambia
- ❑ camellia sinensis
- ❑ Camila
- ❑ Campath
- ❑ Campho-Phenique
- ❑ camphotamide
- ❑ Campral
- ❑ Camptosar
- ❑ camylofine
- ❑ canakinumab
- ❑ Canasa
- ❑ Cancidas
- ❑ candesartan cilexetil
- ❑ Canesten
- ❑ Cankaid
- ❑ cannabidiol
- ❑ cannabinoid
- ❑ cannabinol
- ❑ cannabis sativa
- ❑ Cantil
- ❑ Capastat
- ❑ capecitabine
- ❑ Capex
- ❑ Capoten
- ❑ Capozide
- ❑ Caprelsa
- ❑ capreomycin
- ❑ capryloyl glycine

C

- capsaicin
- capsicum oleoresin
- Captopen
- Captopril
- Captozide
- Capzasin-HP
- Captique
- captodiame
- captopril
- Carac cream
- Carafate
- Carbacel
- carbachol
- Carbaglu
- carbamazepine
- carbamide peroxide
- Carbamine
- Carbatrol
- carbazochrome
- Carb Cutter
- carbenicillin
- carbetapentane
- Carbex
- carbidopa/levodopa
- carbimazole
- carbinoxamine
- carbol-fuchsin paint
- carbolic acid
- carbonic anhydrase inhibitor
- carboplatin
- Carboprost
- Carboptic
- carfilzomib
- Cardene
- Cardilate
- Cardio Essentials
- CardioGen 82
- cardioplegic solution

C

- Cardioquin
- CardioTec Kit
- Cardiotropin
- Cardizem
- Cardura
- carglumic acid
- carisbamate
- carisoprodol
- Carlesta
- Carmex
- carmustine
- Carnitor
- carotenoid
- carphenazine
- Cartelol
- Cartia XT
- Carticel
- Cartrol
- carvedilol
- casanthranol
- cascara sagrada
- Casodex
- caspofungin
- Castiva Arthritis
- castor oil
- Castoria
- Cataflam
- Catapres
- Catapres-TTS
- Catarase
- Catasod-Ocuxtra
- Cathflo Activase
- Catrix
- Caverject
- Cayston
- Ceclor
- Cedax
- CeeNU

C

- ❏ cefaclor
- ❏ cefadroxil monohydrate
- ❏ cefamandole naftate
- ❏ cefazolin
- ❏ cefdinir
- ❏ cefditoren pivoxil
- ❏ cefepime
- ❏ Cefixime
- ❏ Cefizox
- ❏ cefmetazole
- ❏ Cefobid
- ❏ Cefol Filmtab
- ❏ cefonicid
- ❏ cefoperazone
- ❏ Cefotan
- ❏ cefotaxime
- ❏ Cefotetan
- ❏ cefoxitin
- ❏ cefpodoxime
- ❏ cefprozil
- ❏ ceftaroline fosamil
- ❏ ceftazidime
- ❏ ceftibuten
- ❏ Ceftin
- ❏ ceftizoxime
- ❏ Ceftobiprole
- ❏ ceftriaxone
- ❏ cefuroxime
- ❏ cefuroxime axetil
- ❏ Cefzil
- ❏ Celebrex
- ❏ celecoxib
- ❏ Celestone Soluspan
- ❏ Celexa
- ❏ Cellasene
- ❏ CellCept
- ❏ Cellegesic
- ❏ Cellulase

C

- ❏ Cellulean
- ❏ cellulose sodium phosphate
- ❏ Celluvisc lubricant
- ❏ Celontin
- ❏ Cel-U-Jec
- ❏ CenDex
- ❏ Cenestin
- ❏ Centruroides
- ❏ Ceo-Two
- ❏ Cepacol
- ❏ cephalexin
- ❏ cephalosporins
- ❏ cephradine
- ❏ Ceplene
- ❏ Ceprotin
- ❏ Ceptaz
- ❏ Cera
- ❏ CeraVe
- ❏ Cerebyx
- ❏ Cerebrex
- ❏ Ceredase
- ❏ Cerezyme
- ❏ cerivastatin
- ❏ Cernevit
- ❏ Cerose-DM
- ❏ Certican
- ❏ Certiva
- ❏ certolizumab pegol
- ❏ Certriad
- ❏ Cerubidine
- ❏ Cerumenex
- ❏ Cervarix
- ❏ Cervidil
- ❏ Cetacaine
- ❏ Cetamide
- ❏ Cetaphil
- ❏ cethromycin
- ❏ cetirizine

C

- ❑ Cetraxal
- ❑ Cetrorelix
- ❑ Cetrotide
- ❑ cetuximab
- ❑ cetyl alcohol
- ❑ cevimeline
- ❑ Chantix
- ❑ ChapStick
- ❑ charcoal
- ❑ CharcoCaps
- ❑ Chaser Plus
- ❑ Chemet
- ❑ Chenodiol
- ❑ Cheracol
- ❑ Chibroxin
- ❑ ChiRhoStim
- ❑ Chirocaine
- ❑ Chitosan
- ❑ Chlor-3
- ❑ Chloracol
- ❑ chloral hydrate
- ❑ chlorambucil
- ❑ chloramphenicol
- ❑ Chloraseptic
- ❑ chlorcyclizine
- ❑ chlordiazepoxide
- ❑ Chloresium
- ❑ chlorhexidine
- ❑ chlormezanone
- ❑ chloroethane
- ❑ Chlorofair
- ❑ chloroform
- ❑ Chloromycetin
- ❑ chlorophyllin
- ❑ chloroprocaine
- ❑ Chloroptic
- ❑ chloroquine
- ❑ chlorothiazide

C

- ❑ chloroxylenol
- ❑ chlorpheniramine
- ❑ chlorpheniramine polistirex
- ❑ chlorpromazine
- ❑ chlorpropamide
- ❑ chlorprothixene
- ❑ chlorthalidone
- ❑ Chlor Trimeton
- ❑ chlorzoxazone
- ❑ Chocks vitamins
- ❑ Cholebrine
- ❑ cholecalciferol
- ❑ Choledyl
- ❑ ChoLessen
- ❑ Cholestaid
- ❑ Cholesteryl
- ❑ Cholestin
- ❑ cholestyramine
- ❑ choline bitartrate
- ❑ choline magnesium
- ❑ Cholografin
- ❑ Cholybar
- ❑ chondroitin sulfate
- ❑ Chooz
- ❑ choriogonadotropin
- ❑ chorionic gonadotropin
- ❑ Chromagen Forte
- ❑ Chroma Slim
- ❑ chromic chloride
- ❑ chromium picolinate
- ❑ chymotrypsin
- ❑ Cialis
- ❑ Cica-Care
- ❑ ciclesonide
- ❑ ciclopirox
- ❑ cidofovir
- ❑ Cilastin
- ❑ cilostazol

C

- ❑ Ciloxan
- ❑ Ciltyri
- ❑ cimetidine
- ❑ Cimzia
- ❑ cinacalcet
- ❑ Cinobac
- ❑ Cinoxacin
- ❑ Cinryze
- ❑ Cipro
- ❑ Cipro XR
- ❑ Ciprodex
- ❑ ciprofloxacin
- ❑ cisapride
- ❑ cisatracurium besylate
- ❑ cisplatin
- ❑ Cis-Pyro Kit
- ❑ citalopram hydrobromide
- ❑ Citracal
- ❑ CitraNatal
- ❑ citric acid
- ❑ citrocarbonate
- ❑ Citrolith
- ❑ Citrucel
- ❑ civamide
- ❑ Civanex
- ❑ cladribine
- ❑ Claforan
- ❑ Claravis
- ❑ Clarinex
- ❑ Clarinex-D
- ❑ Claripel
- ❑ clarithromycin
- ❑ Claritin
- ❑ Claritin-D
- ❑ clavulanate
- ❑ Clean & Clear
- ❑ Clear Care
- ❑ Clear Eyes

C

- ❑ Clearasil
- ❑ Clear Away
- ❑ clemastine fumarate
- ❑ Clenia
- ❑ Cleocin
- ❑ clevidipine
- ❑ Cleviprex
- ❑ Clidinium
- ❑ Climara
- ❑ Climara Pro
- ❑ Clinac
- ❑ Clinda-Derm
- ❑ Clindagel
- ❑ clindamycin
- ❑ clindamycin hydrochloride
- ❑ clindamycin phosphate
- ❑ Clindesse
- ❑ Clindets Pledgets
- ❑ Clindex
- ❑ Clinimix
- ❑ Clinoril
- ❑ Clinoxide
- ❑ Clioquinol
- ❑ clobazam
- ❑ clobetasol
- ❑ clobetasol propionate
- ❑ Clobevate
- ❑ Clobex
- ❑ clocortolone pivalate
- ❑ clofarabine
- ❑ Clolar
- ❑ Clocream
- ❑ Cloderm
- ❑ Clofazimine
- ❑ clofibrate
- ❑ Clomid
- ❑ clomiphene
- ❑ clomipramine

C

- clonazepam
- Clonicel
- clonidine
- clonidine hydrochloride
- clopidogrel
- clorazepate
- Clorpactin WCS
- Clorpactin WES 90
- Clorpres
- clostridium
- clotrimazole
- cloxacillin
- Cloxapen
- clozapine
- Clozaril
- CM Plex
- CMV-IGIV
- Coartem
- cobicistat
- Cobroxin
- cod liver oil
- Codamine
- codeine
- Codeprex
- Codiclear DH
- Codimal DM
- Codrix
- Coenzyme Q-10
- Cogentin
- Cognex
- Colace
- Colazal
- ColBENEMID
- colchicine
- Colcrys
- Coldcalm
- Cold-EEZE
- colesevelam

C

- Colestid
- colestipol
- colfosceril
- colistimethate
- colistin sulfate
- collagenase
- collagenase clostridium histolyticum
- Collyrium
- Colocort
- Colon Health
- Colonaide
- Coly-Mycin
- Colyte
- Comax
- Combigan
- CombiPatch
- Combipres
- Combivent
- Combivir
- Combunox
- COMFYDE
- Commit
- Compazine
- Complera
- Complete
- Compound W
- Compro
- Comtan
- Comtrex
- Comvax
- Conceptrol
- Concerta
- Condylox
- Congess
- Congespirin
- conivaptan
- conjugated estrogen
- Connexyn

C

- ❏ Conray
- ❏ Constant-T
- ❏ Contac
- ❏ Contac Cold + Flu
- ❏ Contac-D
- ❏ Contrave
- ❏ Copaxone
- ❏ Copegus
- ❏ copper
- ❏ Coppertone
- ❏ CoQ10
- ❏ Coquinone
- ❏ Coramine
- ❏ Cordarone
- ❏ Cordran
- ❏ cordyceps sinensis
- ❏ Cordymax CS
- ❏ Coreg
- ❏ Corgard
- ❏ Coricidin
- ❏ Coricidin HBP
- ❏ Corifact
- ❏ corium
- ❏ Corlopam
- ❏ cormax
- ❏ Corophyllin
- ❏ Correctol
- ❏ Cortaid
- ❏ Cortane-B Otic
- ❏ Cortef
- ❏ Cortenema
- ❏ Cortic ear drops
- ❏ corticorelin
- ❏ corticotropin
- ❏ Cortifoam
- ❏ cortisol
- ❏ cortisone
- ❏ Cortisporin

- ❏ Cortitrol
- ❏ Cortizone-10
- ❏ Cortone
- ❏ Cortrosyn
- ❏ Corvert
- ❏ CorVue
- ❏ Corzide
- ❏ Corzyme
- ❏ Cosamin
- ❏ Cosmegen
- ❏ CosmoDerm
- ❏ CosmoPlast
- ❏ Cosopt
- ❏ cosyntropin
- ❏ Cotanal
- ❏ Cotara
- ❏ Cotazym
- ❏ Co-trimoxazole
- ❏ CoTylenol
- ❏ Coumadin
- ❏ Covera-HS
- ❏ COX-2 inhibitor
- ❏ Cozaar
- ❏ creatine phosphate
- ❏ Creomulsion
- ❏ Creon
- ❏ Crestor
- ❏ Crinone
- ❏ Crixivan
- ❏ crizotinib
- ❏ Crolom
- ❏ cromolyn sodium
- ❏ Cromoptic
- ❏ crotamiton
- ❏ Cruex
- ❏ Cryselle
- ❏ Crystodigin
- ❏ Cubicin

C

- ❑ Culturelle
- ❑ cupric chloride
- ❑ Cuprimine
- ❑ Curad Scar Therapy
- ❑ Cura-Heat
- ❑ CureChrome
- ❑ Curosurf
- ❑ Cutivate
- ❑ Cuyposa
- ❑ CX-516
- ❑ cyanocobalamin
- ❑ Cyanokit
- ❑ Cyclen
- ❑ Cyclessa
- ❑ cyclobarbital
- ❑ cyclobenzaprine
- ❑ Cyclocort
- ❑ Cycloflex
- ❑ Cyclogyl
- ❑ Cyclokapron
- ❑ Cyclomydril
- ❑ cyclopentobarbital
- ❑ cyclopentolate
- ❑ cyclophosphamide
- ❑ cycloserine
- ❑ Cycloset
- ❑ cyclosporine
- ❑ cyclothiazide
- ❑ Cycrin
- ❑ Cylert
- ❑ Cymbalta
- ❑ Cynara-SL
- ❑ cyproheptadine
- ❑ cyproterone
- ❑ Cystadane
- ❑ Cystagon
- ❑ cysteamine
- ❑ Cysto-Conray

C

- ❑ Cystographin
- ❑ Cystospaz
- ❑ Cysview
- ❑ Cytadren
- ❑ cytarabine
- ❑ CytoGam
- ❑ cytomegalovirus vaccine
- ❑ Cytomel
- ❑ Cyto Prep
- ❑ Cytosar-U
- ❑ Cytotec
- ❑ Cytovene
- ❑ Cytoxan

D

- ❑ D-23129
- ❑ dabigatran etexilate
- ❑ D.A. Chewable
- ❑ D.A. Tablets
- ❑ Dacarbazine
- ❑ Daclizumab
- ❑ Dacogen
- ❑ Dacriose
- ❑ dactinomycin
- ❑ Dalalone
- ❑ dalfampridine
- ❑ dalfopristin
- ❑ Dalgin
- ❑ Daliresp
- ❑ Dallergy
- ❑ Dalmane
- ❑ dalteparin sodium
- ❑ Damason-P
- ❑ danazol
- ❑ danaparoid
- ❑ Danocrine

D

- Dantrium
- dantrolene
- Dapagliflozin
- dapiprazole
- dapsone
- Daptacel
- daptomycin
- Daranide
- Daraprim
- darbepoetin alfa
- darifenacin
- Dartal
- darunavir
- Darvocet-A 500
- Darvocet-N
- Darvon
- dasatinib
- Datril
- DaTscan
- daunorubicin
- Daunoxome
- DawnMist
- Daxas
- Daypro
- DayQuil
- Daytrana
- DCF
- DDAVP
- ddC
- Debrox
- Decadron
- Deca-Durabolin
- Decaject
- Decaspray
- decitabine
- Declomycin
- Deconamine
- Deconsal

D

- Decubitene
- Defen-LA
- deferasirox
- deferiprone
- deferoxamine mesylate
- Definity
- Degarelix
- Degest
- dehydro-epiandrosterone
- Delatest injection
- Delatestryl
- delavirdine
- Delcid
- Delestrogen
- Delfen
- Delsym
- Deltasone
- Demadex
- demecarium bromide
- demeclocycline
- Demerol
- Demi-Groton
- Demser
- Demulen
- Denavir
- denileukin diftitox
- Denorex
- denosumab
- Dentapaine
- DentiPatch
- Dent-Zel-Ite
- Depacon
- Depade
- Depakene
- Depakote
- depAndro injection
- Depen
- DepoCyt

D	D

- ❑ DepoDur
- ❑ DepoFoam
- ❑ Depo-Medrol
- ❑ Depomorphine
- ❑ Deponit
- ❑ Depo Provera
- ❑ depo-sub Q provera
- ❑ Depotest injection
- ❑ Depo-Testosterone
- ❑ deprenyl
- ❑ Derifil
- ❑ Dermacil tape
- ❑ Dermaplast
- ❑ Dermarest
- ❑ Derma-Smoothe
- ❑ Dermatop
- ❑ DermOtic Oil
- ❑ Desenex
- ❑ Desferal
- ❑ desflurane
- ❑ desipramine
- ❑ Desirudin
- ❑ Desitin
- ❑ desloratadine
- ❑ desmopressin
- ❑ Desogen
- ❑ desogestrel
- ❑ Desonate
- ❑ desonide
- ❑ DesOwen
- ❑ desoximetasone
- ❑ Desoxyn
- ❑ Despec
- ❑ Desquam-E
- ❑ desvenlafaxine
- ❑ Desyrel
- ❑ detemir
- ❑ Detrol

- ❑ Detrol LA
- ❑ Devonex
- ❑ Dexacort
- ❑ dexamethasone
- ❑ Dexatrim
- ❑ dexbrompheniramine
- ❑ dexchlorpheniramine
- ❑ Dexedrine
- ❑ DexFerrum
- ❑ Dexilant
- ❑ dexlansoprazole
- ❑ dexmedetomidine
- ❑ dexmethylphenidate
- ❑ Dexone
- ❑ Dexpak
- ❑ dexrazoxane
- ❑ dextran-70
- ❑ dextroamphetamine sulfate
- ❑ dextromethorphan
- ❑ dextrose
- ❑ Dextrostat
- ❑ Dezocine
- ❑ DHA
- ❑ DHE-45
- ❑ DHEA
- ❑ DHS tar shampoo
- ❑ DHT Intensol
- ❑ DiaBeta
- ❑ Diabetic Tussin
- ❑ Diabe-Tuss DM
- ❑ Diabet-X
- ❑ Diabinese
- ❑ Dialose
- ❑ Diamox
- ❑ Diamox Sequels
- ❑ Dianeal
- ❑ Diastat
- ❑ diatrizoate

D

- ❏ diatrizoic acid
- ❏ diazepam
- ❏ diazoxide
- ❏ Dibenzyline
- ❏ DiBromm
- ❏ Dicarbosil
- ❏ dichloralphenazone
- ❏ dichlorphenamide
- ❏ diclofenac epolamine
- ❏ diclofenac potassium
- ❏ diclofenac sodium
- ❏ Dicloxacillin
- ❏ dicyclomine
- ❏ didanosine
- ❏ Didrex
- ❏ Didronel
- ❏ dienestrol
- ❏ dienogest
- ❏ diethylpropion
- ❏ diethylstilbestrol diphosphate
- ❏ difenoxin
- ❏ Differin
- ❏ Diff-Quick Stain
- ❏ Dificid
- ❏ diflorasone
- ❏ Diflucan
- ❏ Diflunisal
- ❏ difluprednate
- ❏ Di-Gel
- ❏ Digibind
- ❏ Digitek
- ❏ digoxin
- ❏ digoxin immune fab
- ❏ dihydrocodeine
- ❏ dihydroergotamine
- ❏ dihydrotachysterol
- ❏ diiodohydroxyquin
- ❏ Dilacor

D

- ❏ Dilantin
- ❏ Dilatrate-SR
- ❏ Dilaudid
- ❏ Dilitia
- ❏ Diltiazem
- ❏ Dilor
- ❏ Diluent
- ❏ dimenhydrinate
- ❏ Dimetane-DX
- ❏ Dimetapp
- ❏ dimethicone
- ❏ dimethyl sulfoxide
- ❏ Dinate
- ❏ dinoprostone
- ❏ dioctyl sodium
- ❏ DioMedicone
- ❏ Diovan
- ❏ dioxybenzone
- ❏ Dipentum
- ❏ diphenhydramine
- ❏ diphenidol
- ❏ diphenoxylate
- ❏ diphenylhydantoin
- ❏ diphtheria CRM
- ❏ Dipivefrin
- ❏ dipotassium phosphate
- ❏ Diprivan
- ❏ Diprolene
- ❏ Diprosone
- ❏ dipyridamole
- ❏ diquafosol tetrasodium
- ❏ dirithromycin
- ❏ Disalcid
- ❏ Dismutax
- ❏ Disobrom
- ❏ disodium phosphate
- ❏ disopyramide phosphate
- ❏ Disotate

D

- ❑ DisperMox
- ❑ disulfiram
- ❑ Ditropan
- ❑ Ditropan-XL
- ❑ Diucardin
- ❑ Diuchlor
- ❑ Diulo
- ❑ Diupres
- ❑ Diurex
- ❑ Diuril
- ❑ divalproex sodium
- ❑ Divigel
- ❑ DMARDS
- ❑ DML
- ❑ DMSO
- ❑ Doan's
- ❑ Dobutamine
- ❑ Dobutrex
- ❑ docetaxel
- ❑ docosahexaenoic acid
- ❑ docusate sodium
- ❑ Docusol
- ❑ Dofetilide
- ❑ dolasetron mesylate
- ❑ Dolobid
- ❑ Dolophine
- ❑ Dolorac
- ❑ Domeboro
- ❑ Donatussin
- ❑ donepezil
- ❑ Dong Quai
- ❑ Donnagel
- ❑ Donnatal
- ❑ Donnazyme
- ❑ Dopamine
- ❑ Dopram
- ❑ Doral
- ❑ Dorbane

D

- ❑ Dorbantyl
- ❑ Doribax
- ❑ Doriden
- ❑ doripenem
- ❑ dornase alfa
- ❑ Doryx
- ❑ dorzolamide
- ❑ Dosaflex
- ❑ Dostinex
- ❑ DoubleCap
- ❑ Doubtrex
- ❑ Dovonex
- ❑ doxacurium
- ❑ doxapram
- ❑ doxazosin
- ❑ doxepin
- ❑ doxercalciferol
- ❑ Doxidan
- ❑ Doxil
- ❑ doxorubicin
- ❑ Doxy 100
- ❑ doxychel hyclate
- ❑ doxycycline calcium
- ❑ doxycycline hyclate
- ❑ doxycycline monohydrate
- ❑ doxylamine succinate
- ❑ Dr. Scholl's
- ❑ Drabinol
- ❑ Dramamine
- ❑ Dramanate
- ❑ Drinalfa
- ❑ Dristan
- ❑ Drithrocreme
- ❑ Drixoral
- ❑ Dronabinol
- ❑ dronedarone
- ❑ Droperidol
- ❑ drospirenone

D

- ❑ Drotrecogin Alfa
- ❑ Droxia
- ❑ droxidopa
- ❑ Drysol
- ❑ Dryvax
- ❑ DTIC-Dome
- ❑ Duac
- ❑ Duagen
- ❑ Duet Stuartnatal
- ❑ Duetact
- ❑ Duexa
- ❑ Duexis
- ❑ Dulcodos
- ❑ Dulcolax
- ❑ Dulera
- ❑ duloxetine
- ❑ DuoFilm
- ❑ Duo-Medihaler
- ❑ DuoNeb
- ❑ DuoVisc
- ❑ Duphalic
- ❑ Duracef
- ❑ Duraclon
- ❑ Duract
- ❑ Duradrin
- ❑ Duragesic
- ❑ Dura-Gest
- ❑ Duramorph
- ❑ Duranest
- ❑ Duraphyl
- ❑ Dura-Tap/PD
- ❑ Duratest
- ❑ Durathate
- ❑ Duratuss
- ❑ Dura-Vent
- ❑ Durezol
- ❑ Duricef
- ❑ dutasteride

D

- ❑ DX-88
- ❑ Dyazide
- ❑ Dyclone
- ❑ dyclonine
- ❑ Dyflex
- ❑ Dylix
- ❑ Dyloject
- ❑ Dymelor
- ❑ Dymenate
- ❑ Dynabac
- ❑ Dynacin
- ❑ Dynacirc
- ❑ Dynapen
- ❑ dyphylline
- ❑ Dyrenium
- ❑ Dysport
- ❑ Dytuss

E

- ❑ E2F Decoy
- ❑ EAS Thermo DynamX
- ❑ Easprin
- ❑ Easypod
- ❑ E-Carpine
- ❑ ecallantide
- ❑ Echinacea
- ❑ Echodide
- ❑ echothiophate iodide
- ❑ EC-Naprosyn
- ❑ econazole
- ❑ Econochlor
- ❑ Econopred
- ❑ Ecostatin
- ❑ Ecotrin
- ❑ eculizumab
- ❑ Edarbi

E

- Edecrin
- EdemeX
- edetate disodium
- Edex
- Edluar
- edrophonium
- EDTA
- Edurant
- E.E.S.
- Efacor
- efalizumab
- efavirenz
- Effexor XR
- Effient
- eflornithine
- Efricel
- Efroxine
- Efudex
- E-Gems
- Egrifta
- eicosapentaenoic acid
- ELA-Max
- Elaprase
- Elavil
- Eldepryl
- Eldercaps
- Eldertonic
- Eldopaque
- Eldoquin
- Elecare
- Elestat
- Elestrin
- Eletone cream
- eletriptan
- Elevess
- Elexon
- Elidel cream
- Eligard

E

- Elimite
- Elitek
- Elixicon
- Elixomin
- Elixophyllin
- ElixSure
- ella
- Ellence
- Elmiron
- Elocon
- Eloxatin
- Elspar
- eltrombopag
- elvitegravir
- Emadine
- Embeda
- Embeline
- Embrex 600
- Emcodeine
- Emcyt
- Emdogain
- emedastine
- Emend
- Emergen-C
- Emetrol
- Emgel
- Eminase
- EMLA anesthetic disc
- Empirin
- Emsam
- emtricitabine
- Emtriva
- E-Mycin
- Enablex
- enalapril
- enalaprilat
- Enbrel
- Encainide

E	E

- Endal-HD
- Endantadine
- Endeavor
- Endocet
- Endodan
- Endometrin
- Endrate
- Enduron
- Enecat
- Enfamil Natalins RX
- enflurane
- enfuvirtide
- Engerix-B
- Enhanze SC
- Enjuvia
- Enlon
- Enoxacin
- enoxaparin
- Enpresse
- entacapone
- entecavir
- Entereg
- Enteryx
- Entex
- Entocort
- Entrobar
- ENTSOL
- Enydrial
- Enzyte
- Eovist
- EPA
- Ephedra
- ephedrine
- Epi-C
- Epiduo
- Epifoam
- Epifrin

- E-Pilo
- Epimorph
- Epinal
- epinastine hydrochloride
- epinephrine
- EpiPen Auto-Injector
- EpiPen Jr
- epirubicin
- Epitol
- Epitope
- Epitrate
- Epivir
- Epivir-HBV
- eplerenone
- eplivanserin
- Epoetin Alfa
- Epogen
- epolamine
- epoprostenol
- Epothilone
- Eppy
- epratuzumab
- Eprex
- eprosartan mesylate
- eptifibatide
- Epzicom
- Equagesic
- Equalactin
- Equanil
- Equetro
- Eraxis
- Erbitux
- Ercaf
- Ergamisol
- ergocalciferol
- ergolid mesylate
- Ergomar

E	E

- ❑ ergonovine
- ❑ ergotamine
- ❑ Ergotrate Maleate
- ❑ eribulin mesylate
- ❑ erlotinib
- ❑ Errin
- ❑ Ertaczo
- ❑ ertapenem
- ❑ Erwinase
- ❑ ERYC
- ❑ Erycette
- ❑ Erygel
- ❑ Ery-Max
- ❑ Eryped
- ❑ Ery-Tab
- ❑ Erythrocin
- ❑ erythromycin ethylsuccinate
- ❑ erythropoietin
- ❑ Eryzole
- ❑ Esbriet
- ❑ escitalopram oxalate
- ❑ Esclim
- ❑ Eserin
- ❑ Esgic
- ❑ Esidrix
- ❑ Esimil
- ❑ Eskalith
- ❑ eslicarbazepine acetate
- ❑ esmolol
- ❑ esomeprazole
- ❑ esomeprazole magnesium
- ❑ Essiac tea
- ❑ Essure
- ❑ estazolam
- ❑ esterase
- ❑ Estinyl
- ❑ Estorra
- ❑ Estrace

- ❑ Estraderm
- ❑ estradiol
- ❑ estradiol acetate
- ❑ estradiol cypionate
- ❑ estradiol valerate
- ❑ estramustine phosphate
- ❑ Estratab
- ❑ Estratest
- ❑ Estratest H.S.
- ❑ Estrin-D
- ❑ ESTRING vaginal ring
- ❑ Estrocare
- ❑ EstroGel
- ❑ estrogen
- ❑ estrogen, conjugated
- ❑ estrogen, esterified
- ❑ estropipate
- ❑ Estrasorb
- ❑ Estrostep 21
- ❑ Estrostep FE
- ❑ eszopiclone
- ❑ etanercept
- ❑ ethacrynate sodium
- ❑ ethacrynic acid
- ❑ ethambutol
- ❑ Ethamolin
- ❑ ethanolamine oleate
- ❑ ethchlorvynol
- ❑ ether
- ❑ ethinyl estradiol
- ❑ ethiodized oil
- ❑ Ethiodol
- ❑ ethionamide
- ❑ Ethmozine
- ❑ ethosuximide
- ❑ Ethrane
- ❑ ethyl
- ❑ ethyl aminobenzoate

E

- ❏ ethylbenztropine
- ❏ ethyl chloride
- ❏ ethynodiol diacetate
- ❏ Ethyol
- ❏ etidocaine
- ❏ etidronate disodium
- ❏ etodolac
- ❏ etonogestrel
- ❏ Etopophos
- ❏ etoposide
- ❏ etozolin
- ❏ Etrafon
- ❏ etravirine
- ❏ etretinate
- ❏ ETS
- ❏ eucalyptus
- ❏ Eucerin
- ❏ Eugenol
- ❏ Euglucon
- ❏ Eulexin
- ❏ Eurax
- ❏ Evac-Q-Kwik
- ❏ Evac
- ❏ Evactol
- ❏ Evamist
- ❏ Evercleanse
- ❏ everolimus
- ❏ Everone
- ❏ Evista
- ❏ Evithrom
- ❏ Evoclin
- ❏ Evolence
- ❏ Evoxac
- ❏ EX101
- ❏ Exalgo
- ❏ Exalgo ER
- ❏ Exanta
- ❏ Excedrin
- ❏ Excedrin Quicktabs

E

- ❏ Exelbine
- ❏ Exelon
- ❏ Exemestane
- ❏ exenatide
- ❏ exendin-4
- ❏ Exforge
- ❏ Exforge HCT
- ❏ Exgest
- ❏ Exisulind
- ❏ Exjade
- ❏ Ex-Lax
- ❏ Exna
- ❏ Exosurf
- ❏ Exparel
- ❏ Exsel
- ❏ Extavia
- ❏ Extendryl
- ❏ Extina
- ❏ Extraneal
- ❏ Extrasorb
- ❏ Exubera
- ❏ Eyesine
- ❏ Eye Stream
- ❏ Eylea
- ❏ EZ-Char
- ❏ ezetimibe
- ❏ EZ Med Test
- ❏ ezogabine

F

- ❏ Fablyn
- ❏ Fabrazyme
- ❏ Factive
- ❏ factor IX
- ❏ factor XIII
- ❏ Factrel
- ❏ famciclovir

F

- famotidine
- Fampridine-SR
- Famvir
- Fanapt
- Fansidar
- Fareston
- Faslodex
- Fastin
- fat emulsions
- FazaClo
- FDS feminine spray
- febuxostat
- FEIBA VH
- Felbamate
- Felbatol
- Feldene
- felodipine
- Femara
- Fem-Cap
- FemCare
- Femcet
- Femcon FE
- Femepizole
- Femhrt
- Femizole
- Fempatch
- Femring
- Femstat
- Femtrace
- Fenesin
- fenofibrate
- fenofibric
- Fenoglide
- fenoldopam
- fenoprofen
- Fen-Phen
- fentanyl
- Fentora

F

- Feosol
- Feraheme
- Fero-Folic
- Fero-Grad
- Ferralet
- Ferriprox
- Ferrlecit
- ferrous fumarate
- ferrous gluconate
- ferrous sulfate
- Fertinex
- ferumoxytol
- fesoterodine fumarate
- Fe-Tinic
- Fetrin
- fexofenadine
- fiber
- Fiber Choice
- FiberCon
- Fibrinase
- Fibrinogen
- fidaxomicin
- Filbanserin
- fibrin sealant
- filgrastim
- Finacea
- finasteride
- Finevin cream
- fingolimod
- Fioricet
- Fiorinal
- Fiorpap
- Fiortal
- Firazyr
- Flagyl
- flavocoxid
- flavoxate
- Flebogamma

F

- ❏ flecainide
- ❏ Flector
- ❏ Fleet Anorectal
- ❏ Fleet Babylax
- ❏ Fleet Bisacodyl
- ❏ Fleet Enema
- ❏ Fleet Pedia-Lax
- ❏ Fleet Phospho-Soda
- ❏ Fletcher's Castoria
- ❏ Flex-a-min
- ❏ Flexbumin
- ❏ Flexeril
- ❏ Flexitol
- ❏ Flexitol Blistop
- ❏ Flexoject
- ❏ florbetapir F 18
- ❏ Flolan
- ❏ Flomax
- ❏ Flonase
- ❏ Flo-Pred
- ❏ Florastor
- ❏ Florical
- ❏ Florinef
- ❏ Florone
- ❏ Floropryl
- ❏ Florvite
- ❏ Flovent
- ❏ Flovent Diskus
- ❏ Floxin
- ❏ floxuridine
- ❏ Fluarix
- ❏ Fluclox
- ❏ fluconazole
- ❏ flucytosine
- ❏ Fludara
- ❏ fludarabine
- ❏ fludeoxyglucose F-18
- ❏ fludrocortisones

F

- ❏ FluLaval
- ❏ Flumadine
- ❏ flumazenil
- ❏ FluMist
- ❏ flunisolide
- ❏ flunitrazepam
- ❏ fluocinolone
- ❏ fluocinonide
- ❏ Fluogen
- ❏ Fluonid
- ❏ Fluoracaine
- ❏ fluorescein
- ❏ Fluorescite
- ❏ Fluoreseptic
- ❏ Fluorets
- ❏ Flouri-Methane
- ❏ fluorometholone
- ❏ Fluoroplex
- ❏ fluoroquinolone
- ❏ fluorouracil
- ❏ Fluothane
- ❏ fluoxetine
- ❏ fluoxymesterone
- ❏ fluphenazine
- ❏ flurazepam
- ❏ flurbiprofen
- ❏ Fluress
- ❏ Fluro-Ethyl
- ❏ FluShield
- ❏ fluspirilene
- ❏ fluticasone
- ❏ fluticasone furoate
- ❏ fluticasone propionate
- ❏ flutamide
- ❏ Flutiform
- ❏ fluvastatin
- ❏ Fluvirin
- ❏ fluvoxamine

F

- Fluxid
- Fluzone
- FML
- Focalin
- Folex
- Folgard
- folic acid
- folinic acid
- Follistim
- Follistim/Antagon Kit
- follitropin alfa
- follitropin beta
- Folotyn
- Folvite
- fomepizole
- Fomivirsen
- Fondaparinux sodium
- Foradil
- Forane
- Formadon
- formaldehyde
- Formalin
- formoterol fumarate
- formoterol fumarate dihydrate
- Fortamet
- Fortaz
- Forteo
- Fortesta
- Fortical
- Fortigel
- Fortovase
- Fosamax
- fosamprenavir
- fosaprepitant dimeglumine
- foscarnet
- Foscavir
- fosfomycin

F

- Fosfree
- fosinopril
- fosphenytoin
- fospropofol
- Fosrenol
- Fosteum
- Fo-Ti
- Fototar
- Fragmin
- Framycetin
- FreAmine
- FreeLax
- Frova
- frovatriptan succinate
- FTY720
- FUDR
- Ful-Glo
- fulvestrant
- Fulvicin
- Fumatinic
- Funduscein
- FungiCare
- FungiClear
- FungiCure
- Fungizone
- Fungoid creme
- Furacin
- Furadantin
- Furane
- furazolidone
- Furosemide
- Furoxone
- Fusilev
- Fusion
- fusion inhibitors
- Fuzeon

G

- ❑ gaba analog
- ❑ gabapentin
- ❑ gabapentin enacarbil
- ❑ Gabitril
- ❑ Gablofen
- ❑ Gadavist
- ❑ gadobutrol
- ❑ Gadodiamide
- ❑ gadofosveset
- ❑ gadolinium
- ❑ gadoteridol
- ❑ gadoversetamide
- ❑ gadoxetate
- ❑ galantamine
- ❑ gallamine triethiodide
- ❑ gallium nitrate
- ❑ galsulfase
- ❑ Galzin
- ❑ Gamimune
- ❑ gamma hydroxybutryic acid
- ❑ Gammagard
- ❑ Gammar-P
- ❑ gamma vinyl-GABA
- ❑ Gamunex
- ❑ Gamunex-C
- ❑ ganciclovir
- ❑ Ganirelix
- ❑ Ganite
- ❑ ganoderma lucinum
- ❑ Gantanol
- ❑ Gantrisin
- ❑ Garamycin
- ❑ Gardasil
- ❑ Garnier
- ❑ GasAid
- ❑ Gastrocrom
- ❑ Gastrografin
- ❑ GastroMark

G

- ❑ Gastroview
- ❑ Gas-X
- ❑ gatifloxacin
- ❑ Gattex
- ❑ Gaviscon
- ❑ GBH
- ❑ Gebauer's ethyl chloride
- ❑ Gefitinib
- ❑ Gelcid
- ❑ Gelnique
- ❑ Gel-Ose
- ❑ Gelpirin
- ❑ Gelusil
- ❑ gemcitabine
- ❑ gemfibrozil
- ❑ gemifloxacin mesylate
- ❑ gemtuzumab
- ❑ Gemzar
- ❑ Genapax
- ❑ Genasense
- ❑ Gencaro
- ❑ GenCept
- ❑ GenESA
- ❑ Gen-Glybe
- ❑ Gengraf
- ❑ genistein aglycone
- ❑ Genoptic
- ❑ Genora
- ❑ Genotropin
- ❑ Gentak
- ❑ Gentamicin
- ❑ GenTeal
- ❑ gentian violet
- ❑ Gentlax
- ❑ Gentran 40
- ❑ Gen-Xene
- ❑ genzyme
- ❑ Geocillin

G

- Geodon
- Geopen
- Geref
- Gerimed
- Geriplex
- Geritol
- Geroton
- Gero-Vita
- Gestiva
- Gevrabon
- Gevral
- GHB
- Gilenya
- Gillette
- ginkgo biloba
- Ginkoba
- Ginkogin
- ginseng
- Glandosane
- Glassia
- glatiramer
- Glaucofit
- Glaucon
- Glauma
- Gleevec
- Gliadel
- glimepiride
- glipizide
- globulin
- Glofil-125
- Gluca-Balance
- GlucaGen
- Glucagon [rDNA origin]
- Glucamide
- Glucerna
- glucocerebrosidase
- glucono-delta lactone

G

- Glucophage
- glucosamine sulfate
- glucose oxidase
- glucose polymer
- Glucotrol
- Glucovance
- glulisine
- Glumetza
- Glusamin
- glutamine
- glutathione
- Glutofac
- Glutose
- glyburide
- glycerin
- glyceryl guaiacolate
- glyceryl trinitrate
- glycine
- glycopyrrolate
- glycyrrhetinic acid
- Glynase
- Glynase Prestab
- Gly-Oxide
- Glyquin cream
- Glysenid
- Glyset
- Glyvic
- G-mycetin
- Gold Bond
- gold sodium thiomalate
- golimumab
- GoLYTELY
- gonadorelin
- gonadotropin
- Gonak
- Gonal-F
- Gordochom

G

- ❑ goserelin acetate
- ❑ Gralise
- ❑ gramicidin
- ❑ granisetron
- ❑ Granulex
- ❑ Gravol
- ❑ grepafloxacin
- ❑ Grifulvin V
- ❑ Grisactin
- ❑ griseofulvin
- ❑ Gris-Peg
- ❑ Guaifed
- ❑ guaifenesin
- ❑ guaifenex
- ❑ Guaimax
- ❑ Guai-Vent/PSE
- ❑ guanabenz
- ❑ Guanadrel
- ❑ Guanethidine
- ❑ guanfacine
- ❑ Guanidine
- ❑ Guayanesin
- ❑ guiatuss
- ❑ GVG
- ❑ Gynazole
- ❑ Gyne-Lotrimin
- ❑ Gyne-Trosyd
- ❑ Gynix
- ❑ Gynodiol
- ❑ Gynol II

H

- ❑ H1N1
- ❑ H5N1
- ❑ Habitrol
- ❑ haemophilus beta

H

- ❑ Halaven
- ❑ halcinonide
- ❑ Halcion
- ❑ Haldol
- ❑ Haley's M-O
- ❑ Halfan
- ❑ HalfLytely
- ❑ Halfprin
- ❑ halobetasol propionate
- ❑ halofantrine
- ❑ halog
- ❑ haloperidol
- ❑ Halotestin
- ❑ Halothane
- ❑ Halotussin AC syrup
- ❑ Havrix
- ❑ hawafena
- ❑ Hawaiian Tropic
- ❑ H-BIG
- ❑ HD 85
- ❑ HD 200 Plus
- ❑ Head & Shoulders
- ❑ Head On
- ❑ Healthprin
- ❑ Hectorol
- ❑ Heet
- ❑ Helicosol
- ❑ Helidac therapy
- ❑ Helixate
- ❑ Helixate FS
- ❑ Helizide
- ❑ Hemabate
- ❑ Hemaspan
- ❑ Hematide
- ❑ hemin
- ❑ Hemocyte
- ❑ Hemofil

H

- ❏ Hemorid
- ❏ Hemril suppositories
- ❏ Hemspray
- ❏ HepaGam B
- ❏ Hepalean
- ❏ Heparin
- ❏ Heparine
- ❏ HepatAmine
- ❏ Hep-B-Gammagee
- ❏ Hep-Forte
- ❏ Hepsera
- ❏ heptabarb
- ❏ Herceptin
- ❏ Herpecin-L
- ❏ Herpetrol
- ❏ Herplex
- ❏ HES
- ❏ Hespan
- ❏ Hetastarch
- ❏ Hexabrix
- ❏ Hexadrol
- ❏ Hexalen
- ❏ hexaminolevulinate
- ❏ Hexvix
- ❏ Hiberix
- ❏ Hibiclens
- ❏ Hibistat
- ❏ HibTITER
- ❏ Hismanal
- ❏ Histalet
- ❏ Histatrol
- ❏ Histerone
- ❏ Histinex
- ❏ histolyticum
- ❏ histrelin
- ❏ Histussin HC
- ❏ Hivid
- ❏ Hizentra

H

- ❏ HMG-CoA Reductase inhibitor
- ❏ HMS
- ❏ homatropine
- ❏ homocysteine
- ❏ homosalate
- ❏ Honvol
- ❏ Horizant
- ❏ HPA-23
- ❏ H.P. Acthar Gel
- ❏ Humalog Kwikpen
- ❏ Humalog Pen
- ❏ Humate
- ❏ Humate-P
- ❏ Humatrope
- ❏ Humegon
- ❏ Humibid
- ❏ Humira
- ❏ Humorsol
- ❏ Humulin 50/50
- ❏ Humulin 70/30
- ❏ Humulin N
- ❏ Humulin R
- ❏ Hurricaine
- ❏ Hyalgan
- ❏ hyaluronate
- ❏ hyaluronic acid
- ❏ hyaluronidase
- ❏ Hyate
- ❏ Hycamtin
- ❏ HYcet
- ❏ Hycodan
- ❏ Hycomine
- ❏ Hyco-Pap
- ❏ Hycosin
- ❏ Hycotuss
- ❏ Hydeltra
- ❏ Hydeltrasol
- ❏ Hydergine

H

- ❑ hydralazine
- ❑ hydralazine hydrochloride
- ❑ Hydrate
- ❑ Hydra-Zide
- ❑ hydrazine
- ❑ Hydrea
- ❑ Hydrex
- ❑ Hydrisalic gel
- ❑ Hydrisinol creme
- ❑ Hydrocet
- ❑ hydrochlorothiazide
- ❑ Hydrocil
- ❑ hydrochlorothiazide
- ❑ hydrocodone bitartrate
- ❑ hydrocodone polistirex
- ❑ hydrocortis valerate
- ❑ hydrocortisone
- ❑ Hydrocortone
- ❑ Hydro-D
- ❑ HydroDIURIL
- ❑ hydroflumethiazide
- ❑ hydrogen peroxide
- ❑ Hydromax
- ❑ Hydromet
- ❑ hydromorphone
- ❑ Hydropane syrup
- ❑ Hydropres
- ❑ hydroquinone
- ❑ Hydroxatone
- ❑ hydroxocobalamin
- ❑ hydroxocoralamin
- ❑ hydroxychloroquine
- ❑ Hydroxycut
- ❑ hydroxyprogesterone caproate
- ❑ hydroxypropyl
- ❑ hydroxythiohomosildenafil
- ❑ hydroxyurea
- ❑ hydroxyzine pamoate

H

- ❑ Hygroton
- ❑ Hylaform
- ❑ Hylan GF
- ❑ Hylenex
- ❑ Hylorel
- ❑ hyoscine
- ❑ hyoscyamine
- ❑ Hypaque
- ❑ Hypaque-Cysto
- ❑ Hypaquemeglumine
- ❑ Hyperab
- ❑ HyperHep
- ❑ hypericum
- ❑ Hyperstat
- ❑ Hyper-Tet
- ❑ HypoTears
- ❑ HypRho-D
- ❑ Hyrexin-50
- ❑ hypromellose
- ❑ Hyskon
- ❑ Hytakerol
- ❑ Hytone
- ❑ Hytrin
- ❑ Hyzaar

I

- ❑ Iamin
- ❑ ibandronate
- ❑ Iberet-Folic
- ❑ ibritumomab tiuxetan
- ❑ IBU
- ❑ ibuprofen
- ❑ ibuprofen lysine
- ❑ Ibu-Tab
- ❑ Ibutilide
- ❑ icatibant

I

- IC-Green
- ichthammol
- Iclaprim
- Icy Hot
- Idamycin
- idarubicin
- Identi-Dose
- idoxuride
- idursulfase
- IFEX
- IFN-Alpha 2
- Ilaris
- Ifosamide
- Iletin II, Lente
- Iletin II, NPH
- Ilopan
- iloperidone
- Ilosone
- Ilotycin
- Iluvien
- ILX B-12
- Imagent
- imatinib mesylate
- Imdur
- Imferon
- IMGN529
- imidazole
- imiglucerase
- imipenem
- imipenem & cilastatin
- imipramine pamoate
- imiquimod
- Imitrex
- Imivacurium
- ImmuGo
- Immulite
- Immunocal
- ImmunoLin

I

- Immunopro RX
- Imodium
- Imodium A-D
- Imogam
- Imovax
- Implanon
- ImpoAid
- Impregon
- Impruv
- Imulin
- Imuran
- Inapsine
- Incivek
- incobotulinumtoxinA
- Increlex
- indacaterol
- indapamide
- Inderal
- Inderide
- indinavir
- Indiplon
- Indium
- Indocid
- Indocin
- indocyanine green
- indomethacin
- Infanrix
- Infasurf
- InFeD
- Infergen
- Inflamase
- infliximab
- influenza
- Influenza A (H1N1)
- Infufer
- Infumorph
- Infuvite
- Injectafer

I

- ❑ Innofem
- ❑ Innohep
- ❑ Innopran XL
- ❑ Innovar
- ❑ Inocor
- ❑ INOmax
- ❑ inositol
- ❑ INS365
- ❑ Inspra
- ❑ Instat
- ❑ Insulatard
- ❑ insulin
- ❑ insulin aspart protamine
- ❑ insulin detemir
- ❑ insulin glargine
- ❑ insulin glulisine
- ❑ insulin human
- ❑ insulin lispro
- ❑ insulin lispro protamine
- ❑ Intal
- ❑ Integrilin
- ❑ Integrase inhibitors
- ❑ Intelectol
- ❑ Intelence
- ❑ Intensol
- ❑ Interceed [TC7]
- ❑ Interex
- ❑ interferon alfa-2A
- ❑ interferon alfa-2b
- ❑ interferon alfacon
- ❑ interferon alfacon-1
- ❑ interferon alfacon-a
- ❑ interferon alfa-N3
- ❑ interferon beta-1A
- ❑ interferon beta-1B
- ❑ interferon gamma-1B
- ❑ Intergel
- ❑ Interleukin-1

I

- ❑ Intermezzo
- ❑ Intimex
- ❑ Inti-Mist
- ❑ IntraCoil
- ❑ Intralipid 10 %
- ❑ Intrinsa patch
- ❑ Intron
- ❑ Intropaque
- ❑ Intropin
- ❑ Intuniv
- ❑ inulin
- ❑ Invanz
- ❑ Invega
- ❑ Inversine
- ❑ Invirase
- ❑ iobenguane
- ❑ iodine
- ❑ iodoquinol
- ❑ ioflupane
- ❑ iohexol
- ❑ Ionamin
- ❑ Ionil-T
- ❑ Ionsys transdermal
- ❑ Iontophoretic
- ❑ Iopamidol
- ❑ iopanoic acid
- ❑ Iophen
- ❑ Iophylline
- ❑ iopidine
- ❑ iothalamate meglumine
- ❑ iothalamic acid
- ❑ Ioxalan
- ❑ ipecac
- ❑ ipilimumab
- ❑ iPlex
- ❑ IPOL vaccine
- ❑ ipratropium bromide
- ❑ ipriflavone

I

- ❑ Iprivask
- ❑ Ipsatol
- ❑ Iquix
- ❑ irbesartan
- ❑ Ircon
- ❑ Iressa
- ❑ Irigate
- ❑ irinotecan
- ❑ Iromin-G
- ❑ iron
- ❑ iron carbonyl
- ❑ iron dextran
- ❑ iron polysaccharide
- ❑ iron sucrose
- ❑ Ironman
- ❑ Irospan
- ❑ Isatori Lean
- ❑ Iscar Quercus
- ❑ ISDN
- ❑ Isentress
- ❑ Ismelin
- ❑ Ismo
- ❑ isocarboxazid
- ❑ Isoclor
- ❑ isoetharine
- ❑ isoflurane
- ❑ isoflurophate
- ❑ isometheptene mucate
- ❑ isoniazid
- ❑ isopropyl
- ❑ isoproterenol
- ❑ Isoptin SR
- ❑ Isopto Carbachol
- ❑ Isopto Carpine
- ❑ Isopto Eserine
- ❑ Isordil
- ❑ isosorbide
- ❑ isosorbide dinitrate

I

- ❑ isosorbide mononitrate
- ❑ isotretinoin
- ❑ Isovex
- ❑ Isovorin
- ❑ Isovue-128
- ❑ Isovue-200
- ❑ Isovue-300
- ❑ isoxsuprine
- ❑ isradipine
- ❑ Istalol
- ❑ Istodax
- ❑ Isuprel
- ❑ Itch-X
- ❑ itraconazole
- ❑ IV-AAT
- ❑ Ivarest
- ❑ Iveegam
- ❑ ivermectin
- ❑ Ivy-Dry
- ❑ IvyStat!
- ❑ ixabepilone
- ❑ Ixempra
- ❑ Ixiaro

J

- ❑ Jadelle
- ❑ Jalyn
- ❑ Jantoven
- ❑ Janumet
- ❑ Januvia
- ❑ Jason
- ❑ Jenest
- ❑ Jergens
- ❑ Je-Vax
- ❑ Jevity-Isotonic liquid
- ❑ JointFlex

J

- ❑ Joint-Ritis
- ❑ Jolivette
- ❑ Junel
- ❑ Juvederm
- ❑ Juvisync
- ❑ JZP-6

K

- ❑ Kabikinase
- ❑ Kadian
- ❑ Kalbitor
- ❑ Kaletra
- ❑ Kalydeco
- ❑ Kanamycin
- ❑ Kank-A
- ❑ Kantrex
- ❑ Kaoelectrolyte
- ❑ Kao-Paverin
- ❑ Kaopectate
- ❑ Kapectolin
- ❑ Kapidex
- ❑ Kariva
- ❑ Karno Life
- ❑ Kasof
- ❑ Kava Kava
- ❑ Kayexalate
- ❑ K-Dur microburst
- ❑ Keflex
- ❑ Keftab
- ❑ Kefurox
- ❑ Kefzol
- ❑ Kemadrin
- ❑ Kemstro
- ❑ Kenacort
- ❑ Kenalog
- ❑ Kepivance

K

- ❑ Keppra
- ❑ Keralyt
- ❑ Kerastick
- ❑ Keri Lotion
- ❑ Kerlone
- ❑ Ketalar
- ❑ Ketamine
- ❑ Ketek
- ❑ ketoconazole
- ❑ ketoprofen
- ❑ ketorolac tromethamine
- ❑ ketotifen
- ❑ Key-Pred SP
- ❑ Kidrolase
- ❑ Kie Syrup
- ❑ Kinerase
- ❑ Kineret
- ❑ Kinevac
- ❑ Kinrix
- ❑ Kionex
- ❑ Kivexa
- ❑ Klaron
- ❑ Klondremul
- ❑ Klonopin
- ❑ K-Lor
- ❑ Klor-Con
- ❑ Klotrix
- ❑ Kneerelief
- ❑ Koate-DVI
- ❑ Koate-HP
- ❑ Kogenate
- ❑ KOH solution
- ❑ Kolantyl
- ❑ Kolephrin
- ❑ Kombiglyze
- ❑ Kondremul
- ❑ Konsyl
- ❑ Konyne

K

- ❑ Koo Sar
- ❑ Kophane
- ❑ Koro-Flex
- ❑ Koromex
- ❑ KP Duty
- ❑ K-Phos
- ❑ Kristalose
- ❑ Kronofed
- ❑ Krystexxa
- ❑ K-Tab
- ❑ Kudrox
- ❑ kunecatechins
- ❑ Kutrase
- ❑ Kuvan
- ❑ Ku-Zyme
- ❑ Kwelcof
- ❑ Kwell
- ❑ KY-Plus
- ❑ Kynapid
- ❑ Kytril

L

- ❑ labetalol
- ❑ Lac-Hydrin
- ❑ Laclotion
- ❑ lacosamide
- ❑ Lacri-Lube
- ❑ Lacrisert
- ❑ Lactaid
- ❑ lactalbumin hydrolysate
- ❑ lactase
- ❑ lactic acid
- ❑ Lacticare
- ❑ Lactinol
- ❑ lactobacillus reuteri
- ❑ Lactocal

L

- ❑ lactulose
- ❑ Lamictal
- ❑ Lamictal XR
- ❑ Lamisil
- ❑ lamivudine
- ❑ lamotrigine
- ❑ Lamprene
- ❑ Lanacane
- ❑ lanolin
- ❑ Lanophyllin
- ❑ Lanoxicaps
- ❑ Lanoxin
- ❑ lanreotide acetate
- ❑ lansoprazole
- ❑ lanthanum carbonate
- ❑ Lantus
- ❑ Lantus SoloStar
- ❑ lapatinib
- ❑ Lariam
- ❑ Laradopa
- ❑ Largactil
- ❑ L-arginine
- ❑ laromustine
- ❑ laronidase
- ❑ Lasix
- ❑ lasofoxifene
- ❑ L-asparaginase
- ❑ Lastacaft
- ❑ Latanoprost
- ❑ Latisse
- ❑ Latuda
- ❑ laViv
- ❑ Laudanum
- ❑ Lanzanda
- ❑ Lazerformaldehyde
- ❑ Lazersporin
- ❑ L-Carnitine
- ❑ L-Cystine

L

❑ Lecithin
❑ Ledercillin
❑ Leena
❑ leflunomide
❑ Legatrin
❑ lenalidomide
❑ Lente Iletin
❑ lepirudin
❑ Leptoprin
❑ lercanidipine
❑ Leritine
❑ Lescol
❑ Lessina
❑ Letairis
❑ letrozole
❑ Leucovorin
❑ Leucovorin rescue
❑ Leukeran
❑ Leukine
❑ Leukotriene
❑ leuprolide
❑ Leustatin
❑ Levadex
❑ levalbuterol
❑ levallorphan
❑ levamisole
❑ Levaquin
❑ Levatol
❑ Levbid
❑ Levemir
❑ levetiracetam
❑ Levitra
❑ Levlen
❑ Levlite
❑ levmetamfetamine
❑ levobetaxolol
❑ levobunolol
❑ levobupivacaine
❑ levocabastine

L

❑ levocarnitine
❑ levocetirizine dihydrochloride
❑ levodopa
❑ Levo-Dromoran
❑ levofloxacin
❑ Levolet
❑ levoleucovorin
❑ levomefolate
❑ levomethadyl acetate
❑ levonorgestrel
❑ Levoprome
❑ Levora
❑ levorphanol
❑ Levo-T
❑ Levothroid
❑ levothyroxine
❑ Levoxyl
❑ Levsin
❑ Levsinex Timecaps
❑ Levulan Kerastick
❑ Lexapro
❑ Lexidronam
❑ Lexiscan
❑ Lexiva
❑ Lexxel
❑ L-glutamic acid
❑ L-glutamine
❑ Lialda
❑ LibiGel
❑ Libra
❑ Librax
❑ Libritabs
❑ Librium
❑ Lidex
❑ lidocaine
❑ Lidoderm patch
❑ lidoflazine
❑ LidoPen Auto-Injector
❑ LidoSite

L

- Lifegenes spray
- Lifepak capsules
- Limbitrol
- Limbrel
- Linaclotide
- linagliptin
- Lincocin
- Lincomycin
- Lindane
- Linezolid
- Linjeta
- Linosamide
- Lioresal
- liothyronine
- Liotrix
- Lipase
- Lipitor
- lipoic acid
- Liposyn
- LipoTrim
- Liprotamase
- Lipsovir
- Liqui-Char
- Liquibeads
- Liquibid
- Liquipake
- Liquipred
- Liquiprin
- liraglutide
- lisdexamfetamine dimesylate
- lisinopril
- lithium carbonate
- lithium citrate
- Lithobid
- Lithonate
- Lithostat
- Lithotabs
- Little Tummys
- Livalo

L

- Livial
- Lixolin
- L.M.X.4 cream
- L.M.X.5 cream
- LMD
- L'OREAL
- LoCholest
- Locoid Lipocreme
- Locteron
- Lodine
- Lodosyn
- Lodox
- Lodoxamide
- Lodoxide
- Lodrane
- Loestrin
- Loestrin 24 Fe
- Lofibra
- loflupane
- Lo Loestrin Fe
- lomefloxacin
- L-O-M Mus softgel
- Lomotil
- lomustine
- Loniten
- Lonox
- Lo/Ovral
- loperamide
- Lopid
- lopinavir
- Lopressor
- Loprox
- Lorabid
- loracarbef
- Loramyc
- loratadine
- lorazepam
- Lorcaserin
- Lorcet

L

- Lorelco
- Lorfan
- Loridine
- Lortab
- losartan
- LoSeasonique
- Lotemax
- Lotensin
- loteprednol
- Lotrel
- Lotrimin
- Lotrisone
- Lotrix
- Lotronex
- lovastatin
- Lovaza
- Lovenox
- Lovpil
- Low-Ogestrel
- loxapine
- Loxitane
- Lozol
- LSAID
- LSD
- lubiprostone
- Lubriderm
- Lubrin
- Lucassin
- Lucentis
- lucinactant
- Ludiomil
- Lufyllin-GG
- lumefantrine
- Lumene
- Lumigan
- Lumizyme
- Lunelle
- Lunesta
- Lupron

L

- lurasidone
- Luride
- Lurline
- Lusedra
- Lustra
- lutein
- Lutera
- Lutrepulse
- lutropin alfa
- Luveniq
- Luveris
- Luvox
- Luxi☐ foam
- LX211
- Lybrel
- lycopene
- LYMErix
- Lymphazurin
- Lypressin
- Lyrica
- lysergic acid diethylamide
- Lysine
- Lysodren
- Lysteda

M

- MAA kit
- Maalox
- Macrobid
- Macrodantin
- macrolide
- Macugen
- Macutein
- mafenide acetate
- Mag-al
- Magan
- Magnaril

M

❑ magnesium
❑ magnesium carbonate
❑ magnesium hydroxide
❑ magnesium oxide
❑ magnesium sulfate
❑ magnesium trisilicate
❑ Magnevist
❑ Magnolax
❑ Magonate
❑ Mag-Ox
❑ Magsal
❑ Magtab SR
❑ ma huang
❑ Maintain
❑ Makena
❑ Malarone
❑ Malathion
❑ Maltsupex
❑ Mandelamine
❑ ManDelay
❑ Mandol
❑ Manerex
❑ Mangafodipir
❑ manganese
❑ Mann-Dino
❑ Mannitol
❑ Mantadil
❑ MAO inhibitor
❑ Maox
❑ maprotiline
❑ maraviroc
❑ Marax
❑ Marblen
❑ Marcaine
❑ MarineOmega
❑ Marinol
❑ Marlyn
❑ Marplan
❑ Marvelon

M

❑ Massengill douche
❑ Masoprocol
❑ MasXtreme
❑ Materna
❑ Matulane
❑ Mavik
❑ Max-Freeze
❑ Maxair Autohaler
❑ Maxalt
❑ Maxalt-MLT
❑ Maxaquin
❑ Maxidex
❑ Maxidone
❑ Maxifed
❑ Maxiflor
❑ Maxipime
❑ Maxitrol
❑ Maxzide
❑ May-Vita
❑ Mazepine
❑ mazindo
❑ MDP Kit
❑ MDR Fitness
❑ Mebaral
❑ mebendazole
❑ mecamylamine
❑ mecasermin
❑ mechlorethamine
❑ Meclan
❑ meclizine
❑ meclofenamate
❑ Meclomen
❑ Mederma
❑ Medifast
❑ Medigesic
❑ Mediplex
❑ Medizym
❑ Medi-Zyme
❑ Medrol

M	M

- ❏ medroxyprogesterone
- ❏ mefenamic acid
- ❏ mefloquine
- ❏ Mefoxin
- ❏ Mega-B
- ❏ Megace
- ❏ Megadose
- ❏ Mega MSM
- ❏ megestrol acetate
- ❏ Melanex
- ❏ melatonin
- ❏ Mellaril
- ❏ meloxicam
- ❏ melphalan
- ❏ MEM 1414
- ❏ memantine
- ❏ Menactra
- ❏ MenACWY-CRM
- ❏ MenHibrix
- ❏ Menest
- ❏ meningococcal conjugate
- ❏ Menocheck
- ❏ Menomune
- ❏ Menostar
- ❏ menotropin
- ❏ Mentax
- ❏ Mentholatum
- ❏ Menveo
- ❏ mepenzolate bromide
- ❏ Mepergan
- ❏ meperidine
- ❏ mephobarbital
- ❏ Mephyton
- ❏ mepivacaine
- ❏ meprobamate
- ❏ Mepron
- ❏ Mequinol
- ❏ mercaptopurine

- ❏ Mercurochrome
- ❏ Meribin
- ❏ Meridia
- ❏ Merlot
- ❏ meropenem
- ❏ Merrem I.V.
- ❏ Mertazapine
- ❏ Merthiolate
- ❏ Meruvax
- ❏ mesalamine
- ❏ mesantoin
- ❏ Mescolor
- ❏ Mesna
- ❏ Mesnex
- ❏ mesoridazine
- ❏ Mestinon
- ❏ Mestranol
- ❏ Metab-O-Fx
- ❏ Metabolife
- ❏ Metadate-CD
- ❏ Metaglip
- ❏ Metahydrin
- ❏ Metamucil
- ❏ metaproterenol
- ❏ metaraminol bitartrate
- ❏ Metastron
- ❏ metaxalone
- ❏ metformin
- ❏ methacholine
- ❏ methadone
- ❏ Methadose
- ❏ methamphetamine
- ❏ methaqualone
- ❏ methazolamide
- ❏ methenamine hippurate
- ❏ methimazole
- ❏ methionine
- ❏ methobarbital

M

- methocarbamol
- methohexital
- Methosalen
- methotrexate
- methoxamine
- methoxsalen
- methoxy polyethylene glycol-epoetin
- methscopolamine
- methsuximide
- methulose
- methyclothiazide
- methyl aminolevulinate
- methylatropine bromide
- methyldopa
- methyldopate
- methylene blue
- methylene trichloride
- methylergonovine
- methyl green
- Methylin
- methylnaltrexone bromide
- methylphenidate
- methylpred
- methylprednisolone
- methyl salicylate
- methyl sulfate
- methyltestosterone
- methylthiouracil
- methyl violet
- methyl xanthine
- methysergide
- Metimyd
- metoclopramide
- metocurine iodide
- metolazone
- metoprolol succinate
- metoprolol tartrate
- Metozolv ODT

M

- Metreleptin
- MetroCream
- Metrodin
- MetroGel
- MetroLotion
- metronidazole
- metropirone
- Metubine
- Metvixia
- metyrapone
- metyrosine
- Mevacor
- mevastatin
- mexiletine
- Mexitil
- Mezlin
- mezlocillin
- MHP TakeOff Hi-Energy
- micafungin
- Miacalcin
- Micanol
- Micardis
- Micatin
- miconazole
- miconazole lauriad
- Micort-HC
- MICRhoGAM
- Micro-K
- Microgestin
- Microgestin Fe
- Micronase
- micronized colestipol
- Micronor
- Microzide
- Midamor
- Midazolam
- midodrine
- Midol

M

- Midrin
- Mifeprex
- mifepristone [RU486]
- Miglitol
- miglustat
- MigraHealth
- Migralam
- Migra Migraine spray
- Migranal
- Milkinol
- Milk of Magnesia
- milnacipran
- Milontin
- Milophene
- milrinone
- Miltown
- Mimyx cream
- minerals
- mineral oil
- Minestrin
- Minipress
- Minitran
- Minit-Rub
- Minizide
- Minocin
- minocycline
- minoxidil
- Mintezole
- Miocel
- Miochol
- Mio-Rel
- Miostat
- Mipomersen
- Mirabegron
- Miracle of Aloe Miracure
- Miradon
- MiraLAX
- Miranel

M

- Mirapex
- Mirapex ER
- Mircera
- Mircette
- Mirena
- mirtazapine
- misoprostol
- Mithracin
- mithramycin
- mitomycin
- mitotane
- mitoxantrone
- Mitozytrex
- MitraFlex
- Mivacron
- mivacurium
- Miveprev
- Mixtard
- M-M-R II
- Moban
- Mobic
- Mobigesic
- Modafinil
- Modane
- Moderil
- ModiCon
- Modrastane
- Moduretic
- moexipril
- Moi-Stir
- Moisturel
- molindone
- mometasone furoate
- mometasone furoate monohydrate
- Monarc-M
- monascus purpuerus went
- Monistat
- Monistat 3

M

- ❑ Monistat 7
- ❑ monoamine oxidase inhibitor
- ❑ monobenzone
- ❑ Monocal
- ❑ Monocid
- ❑ Monoclate-P
- ❑ Monodox
- ❑ monofluorophosphate
- ❑ Monogesic
- ❑ monohydrate
- ❑ Monoket
- ❑ Mononessa
- ❑ Mononine
- ❑ Monopril
- ❑ Mono-Vacc
- ❑ montelukast
- ❑ Monurol
- ❑ moricizine
- ❑ MOPP
- ❑ morphine sulfate
- ❑ morrhuate sodium
- ❑ Motavizumab
- ❑ Motofen
- ❑ Motrin
- ❑ MoviPrep
- ❑ Moxatag
- ❑ MoxDuo IR
- ❑ Moxeza
- ❑ moxifloxacin
- ❑ Moxilin
- ❑ Mozobil
- ❑ M-R VAX
- ❑ MS-325
- ❑ MS Contin
- ❑ MSIR
- ❑ MSM
- ❑ MSTA
- ❑ MT100

M

- ❑ MTS
- ❑ Mucinex
- ❑ Mucinex D
- ❑ Mucinex DM
- ❑ Mucinex Mini-Melts
- ❑ Muco-Fen
- ❑ Mucomyst
- ❑ Mucosil
- ❑ Mudrane
- ❑ Multaq
- ❑ Mumpsvax
- ❑ mupirocin
- ❑ Murine
- ❑ Muro 128
- ❑ Muro Gonio-Gel
- ❑ muromonab-CD3
- ❑ MUSE
- ❑ Mustargen
- ❑ Mutamycin
- ❑ M.V.I.
- ❑ Myambutol
- ❑ Mycamine
- ❑ Mycelex
- ❑ Myclo
- ❑ Mycobutin
- ❑ Mycocide
- ❑ Mycolog
- ❑ mycophenolate mofetil
- ❑ mycophenolic
- ❑ Mycostatin
- ❑ Myerlan
- ❑ Myfortic
- ❑ Mykrox
- ❑ Mylanta
- ❑ Myleran
- ❑ Mylicon
- ❑ Mylotarg
- ❑ Myobloc

M

- ❑ myochrysine
- ❑ Myoflex
- ❑ Myoview
- ❑ Myozyme
- ❑ myrrh
- ❑ Mysoline
- ❑ Mytelase
- ❑ Mytozytrex
- ❑ Mytrate
- ❑ Mytrex
- ❑ M-Zole 3

N

- ❑ NABI-HB
- ❑ nabilone
- ❑ nabumetone
- ❑ nadolol
- ❑ Nadopen
- ❑ Nadostine
- ❑ Nads
- ❑ Nafarelin
- ❑ nafcillin
- ❑ naftifine
- ❑ Naftin
- ❑ Naglazyme
- ❑ Nair
- ❑ nalbuphine
- ❑ Nalex
- ❑ Nalfon
- ❑ nalidixic acid
- ❑ Nallpen
- ❑ nalmefene
- ❑ naloxone
- ❑ naltrexone
- ❑ Namenda
- ❑ nambutone

N

- ❑ nandrolone decanoate
- ❑ naphazoline
- ❑ Naphcon A
- ❑ Naprelan
- ❑ Naprosyn
- ❑ naproxcinod
- ❑ naproxen
- ❑ naproxen sodium
- ❑ Naqua
- ❑ naratriptan
- ❑ Narcan
- ❑ Nardil
- ❑ Naropin
- ❑ Nasacort AQ
- ❑ NasalCrom
- ❑ NasalFent
- ❑ Nasalide
- ❑ Nasarel
- ❑ Nasatab
- ❑ Nascobal
- ❑ Nasonex
- ❑ Natachew
- ❑ Natafort
- ❑ natalizumab
- ❑ natamycin
- ❑ Natazia
- ❑ nateglinide
- ❑ Natrecor
- ❑ Natroba
- ❑ Natrol
- ❑ Natrol CitriMax
- ❑ Nature's Bounty Xtreme Lean
- ❑ Nature-throid
- ❑ Naturetin
- ❑ Nauzene
- ❑ Navane
- ❑ Navelbine
- ❑ Navstel

N

- Nebcin
- Nebido
- nebivolol
- NebuPent
- Necon
- nedocromil
- N.E.E.
- nefazodone
- NegGram
- nelarabine
- nelfinavir
- Nelfon
- Nelova
- Nelulen
- Nembutal
- Neo-Codema
- Neo-Cortef
- Neo-Decadron
- Neo-Delta-Cortef
- Neolax
- Neoloid
- Neo-Medrol
- neomycin
- Neo-Polycin
- NeoProfen
- Neoral
- Neosar
- Neosporin
- neostigmine
- Neo-Synephrine
- NeoTect
- Neothylline
- Neovastat
- Neozin
- nepafenac
- NephrAmine
- Nephro-Calci
- Nephrocaps

N

- Nephro-Fer
- Nephro-Vite Rx
- Nephrox
- Neptazane
- Nesacaine
- nesiritide
- Nestabs CBF
- netilmicin
- Netromycin
- Netupitant
- Neulasta
- Neumega
- Neupogen
- Neupro
- Neuro-Balance
- Neuromins-DHA
- Neurontin
- Neutrexin
- Neutrogena
- Nevanac
- nevirapine
- Nexavar
- Nexium
- Nexterone
- niacin
- niacinamide
- Niacor
- Niaspan
- nicardipine
- NicoDerm CQ
- Nicolar
- Nicomide
- Nicorette gum
- Nicosyn
- Nicotinamide
- nicotine polacrilex
- Nicotinex
- nicotinic acid

N

- ❏ Nicotrol
- ❏ nifedipine
- ❏ Niferex
- ❏ Nilandron
- ❏ nilotinib
- ❏ Nilstat
- ❏ nilutamide
- ❏ Nimbex
- ❏ nimodipine
- ❏ Nimotop
- ❏ Niox
- ❏ Nipent
- ❏ Nipolept
- ❏ Niravam
- ❏ nisoldipine
- ❏ nitazoxanide
- ❏ nitisinone
- ❏ Nitrek
- ❏ Nitro-Bid
- ❏ Nitrodisc
- ❏ Nitro-Dur
- ❏ nitrofurantoin
- ❏ nitrofurazone
- ❏ nitroglycerin
- ❏ Nitrol
- ❏ Nitrolingual Pumpspray
- ❏ NitroMist
- ❏ Nitrostat
- ❏ nitrous oxide
- ❏ Nivea
- ❏ Nix Shampoo
- ❏ nizatidine
- ❏ Nizoral A-D
- ❏ No Doz
- ❏ Noah's Naturals
- ❏ Nolahist
- ❏ Nolamine
- ❏ Nolvadex

N

- ❏ nonoxynol-9
- ❏ NonyX
- ❏ Nora-BE
- ❏ Norcept
- ❏ Norco
- ❏ Norcuron
- ❏ Nordette
- ❏ Norditropin
- ❏ Norel DM
- ❏ Norel SR
- ❏ norelgestromin
- ❏ norethindrone
- ❏ Norflex
- ❏ norfloxacin
- ❏ Norforms
- ❏ Norgesic
- ❏ norgestimate
- ❏ norgestrel
- ❏ Norinyl
- ❏ Noritate
- ❏ Norlestrin
- ❏ Normiflo
- ❏ Normodyne
- ❏ Noroxin
- ❏ Norpace
- ❏ Norplant
- ❏ Norpramin
- ❏ Nor-QD
- ❏ Nortemp
- ❏ Northera
- ❏ Nortrel
- ❏ nortriptyline
- ❏ Norvasc
- ❏ Norvir
- ❏ Novacet
- ❏ Novaldex
- ❏ Novamine
- ❏ Novamoxin

N

- Novantrone
- Novarel
- Novitra
- Novocain
- Novo-Clobazam
- Novolin
- NovoLog
- Novopen
- NovoSeven
- Novo-Thalidone
- Novothyrox
- novotriphyl
- Noxafil
- Noxzema
- NPH Iletin
- Nplate
- NSAID
- NT-Kinase
- NU-Iron
- Nubain
- Nucofed
- Nucynta
- Nuedexta
- NuFill
- Nuflexxa
- NuLev
- Nulojix
- NuLYTLEY
- Numorphan
- Numzident
- Num-Zit-Gel
- Nunaturals LevelRight
- Nupercainal
- Nuromax
- Nutracort
- Nutropin
- Nutropin AQ
- Nutropin Nuspin

N

- Nutropin Pen
- NuvaRing
- Nuvigil
- Nuvion
- Nydrazid
- NyQuil
- Nystatin
- Nystop
- Nytilax
- Nytol

O

- OBEGYN
- Obinex
- oblimersen
- Oby-Cap
- OCC
- Ocean
- Ocella
- Octagam
- octocrylene
- octoxynol-9
- octreotide acetate
- octyl dimethyl
- Ocu-Chlor
- Ocucoat
- Ocufen
- Ocuflox
- OcuFresh
- OcuGuard
- OcuHist
- Ocu-Mycin
- OCuSOFT
- Ocusol
- Ocu-Spor
- Ocusporin

○ ○

- ❑ Ocu-Sul
- ❑ Ocusulf
- ❑ Ocutricin
- ❑ ofatumumab
- ❑ Ofirmev
- ❑ ofloxacin
- ❑ OGEN
- ❑ Ogestrel
- ❑ OKA
- ❑ olanzapine
- ❑ oleandomycin
- ❑ Oleptro
- ❑ olive oil
- ❑ olmesartan medoxomil
- ❑ olopatadine
- ❑ olsalazine
- ❑ Olux Foam
- ❑ Olux-E Foam
- ❑ omacetaxine mepesuccinate
- ❑ Omacor
- ❑ omalizumab
- ❑ Omapro
- ❑ omega-3 acids
- ❑ omega-3 ethyl esters
- ❑ omega-3 polyunsaturates
- ❑ omeprazole
- ❑ Omnaris
- ❑ Omnicef
- ❑ OmniHIB
- ❑ Omnihist
- ❑ Omnipaque
- ❑ Omnipen
- ❑ Omniscan
- ❑ Omnitrope
- ❑ onabotulinumtoxinA
- ❑ Oncaspar
- ❑ Oncolym
- ❑ Oncovin

- ❑ ondansetron
- ❑ One-A-Day Weight Smart
- ❑ Onfi
- ❑ Onglyza
- ❑ On-Q
- ❑ Onrigin
- ❑ Onsolis
- ❑ Ontak
- ❑ Ony-Clear
- ❑ Opana
- ❑ Opana ER
- ❑ Opcon-A
- ❑ Ophthacet
- ❑ Ophthaine
- ❑ Ophthetic
- ❑ Ophthochlor
- ❑ Ophthocort
- ❑ Ophtho-Diprivefrin
- ❑ oprelvekin
- ❑ Optaflu
- ❑ Opticrom
- ❑ Opti-Free
- ❑ OptiGold
- ❑ OptiMark
- ❑ Optimine
- ❑ Optimyd
- ❑ Optipranolol
- ❑ Optiray
- ❑ Optivar
- ❑ Optson
- ❑ Orabase
- ❑ Oracea
- ❑ OraDisc A
- ❑ Oragrafin
- ❑ Orajel
- ❑ Oramorph
- ❑ Orap
- ❑ Oraphen-PD

O

O

- ❑ Orapred
- ❑ Oraqix
- ❑ OraQuick
- ❑ OraSure
- ❑ OraVerse
- ❑ OraVescent Fentanyl
- ❑ Oravig
- ❑ OrCel
- ❑ Orencia
- ❑ Oretic
- ❑ Orex
- ❑ Orfadin
- ❑ Organidin NR
- ❑ Orgaran
- ❑ Orinase
- ❑ Orlaam
- ❑ Orlistat
- ❑ Ornade
- ❑ Ornex
- ❑ orphenadrine
- ❑ orphengesic
- ❑ Ortho-Cept
- ❑ Orthoclone OKT3
- ❑ Ortho-Creme
- ❑ Ortho-Cyclen
- ❑ Ortho-Dienestrol
- ❑ Ortho-Est
- ❑ Ortho-Gynol
- ❑ Ortho Micronor
- ❑ Ortho-Novum
- ❑ Ortho-Prefest
- ❑ Ortho Evra
- ❑ Ortho Tri-Cyclen
- ❑ Ortho Tri-Cyclen Lo
- ❑ Orthovisc
- ❑ Orudis
- ❑ Oruvail
- ❑ Orzel

- ❑ Os-Cal
- ❑ Oscillo
- ❑ Oscillococcinum
- ❑ oseltamivir
- ❑ Osmoglyn
- ❑ OsmoPrep
- ❑ Osteo Bi-Flex
- ❑ OTG
- ❑ Otocain
- ❑ OvaRex
- ❑ Ovcon
- ❑ Ovide
- ❑ Ovidrel
- ❑ Ovocyclin
- ❑ Ovral
- ❑ Ovrette
- ❑ oxacillin
- ❑ Oxaine
- ❑ oxaliplatin
- ❑ Oxandrin
- ❑ oxandrolone
- ❑ oxaprozin
- ❑ Oxazepam
- ❑ oxazolidinone
- ❑ oxcarbazepine
- ❑ Oxecta
- ❑ oxiconazole
- ❑ Oxilan
- ❑ Oxistat
- ❑ Oxsoralen
- ❑ oxtriphylline
- ❑ Oxy
- ❑ oxybenzone
- ❑ oxybutynin chloride
- ❑ oxybutynin hydrochloride
- ❑ oxycodone
- ❑ OxyContin
- ❑ OxyFast

O

- ❑ OxyIR
- ❑ oxymetazoline
- ❑ oxymetholone
- ❑ oxymorphone
- ❑ oxyquinoline
- ❑ Oxyspectro
- ❑ oxytetracycline
- ❑ oxytocin
- ❑ Oxytrol
- ❑ Ozogamicin
- ❑ Ozurdex

P

- ❑ PA-824
- ❑ Pacaps
- ❑ Pacerone
- ❑ paclitaxel
- ❑ Paddock Podofliox
- ❑ padimate
- ❑ Pain Bust
- ❑ PainBust-R
- ❑ PainPatch
- ❑ Palaron
- ❑ palifermin
- ❑ paliperidone
- ❑ palivizumab
- ❑ Palladone
- ❑ Palmatate
- ❑ palonosetron HCl
- ❑ pamabrom
- ❑ Pamelor
- ❑ pamidronate
- ❑ Pamine
- ❑ Pamprin
- ❑ Panafil
- ❑ Panafil SE

P

- ❑ Panalgesic Gold Cream
- ❑ Panax
- ❑ Pancrease MT
- ❑ pancreatin
- ❑ Pancreaze
- ❑ pancrelipase
- ❑ pancuronium bromide
- ❑ Pandel
- ❑ Panglobulin NF
- ❑ Panhematin
- ❑ panitumumab
- ❑ Panmycin
- ❑ PanOxyl
- ❑ Panretin
- ❑ Panthenol
- ❑ pantoprazole
- ❑ pantothenate calcium
- ❑ pantothenic acid
- ❑ Panwarfin
- ❑ papain
- ❑ papaverine
- ❑ papillomavirus
- ❑ para-amino benzoic acid
- ❑ Paradione
- ❑ Paraflex
- ❑ Parafon Forte
- ❑ ParaGard T380 A
- ❑ paraldehyde
- ❑ Paraplatin
- ❑ Parathar
- ❑ Parcopa
- ❑ paregoric
- ❑ Paremyd
- ❑ parepectolin
- ❑ paricalcitol
- ❑ Parlodel
- ❑ Parnate
- ❑ paroxetine

P

- ❑ Paser
- ❑ Patady
- ❑ Patanase
- ❑ Patanol
- ❑ PatentLean
- ❑ Pathiam
- ❑ Pathocil
- ❑ Pavabid
- ❑ Pavulon
- ❑ Paxil
- ❑ Paxil CR
- ❑ Pazo
- ❑ pazopanib
- ❑ PBZ
- ❑ PCE
- ❑ PCP
- ❑ PC Spes
- ❑ PDE5 blocker
- ❑ PediaCare
- ❑ Pediacof
- ❑ Pediaflor
- ❑ Pedia-Lax
- ❑ Pedialyte
- ❑ Pediapred
- ❑ Pediarix
- ❑ PediaSure
- ❑ Pediazole
- ❑ Pedi-Boro Soak Paks
- ❑ Pedi-Dri
- ❑ PediOtic
- ❑ PedvaxHIB
- ❑ PEG-3350
- ❑ pegademase
- ❑ Peganone
- ❑ pegaptanib
- ❑ pegaspargase
- ❑ Pegasys
- ❑ pegfilgrastim

P

- ❑ peginesatide
- ❑ peginterferon
- ❑ peginterferon alfa-2B
- ❑ PEG-Intron
- ❑ pegloticase
- ❑ pegvisomant
- ❑ pemetrexed
- ❑ pemirolast
- ❑ Pemoline
- ❑ penbutolol
- ❑ Pen-Colate
- ❑ penciclovir
- ❑ Penecort
- ❑ Penetrex
- ❑ penicillin
- ❑ penicillin G benzathine
- ❑ penicillin G procaine
- ❑ penicillamine
- ❑ Penlac
- ❑ Pennsaid
- ❑ Pentacel
- ❑ pentagastrin
- ❑ Pentam
- ❑ pentamidine
- ❑ Pentamycetin
- ❑ Pentasa
- ❑ Pentaspan
- ❑ Pentastarch
- ❑ pentazocine
- ❑ Pentetate
- ❑ pentobarbital
- ❑ pentosan polysulfate sodium
- ❑ pentostatin
- ❑ Pentothal, Sodium
- ❑ pentoxifylline
- ❑ Pentoxil
- ❑ Pen-Vee
- ❑ Pep-Back

P	P

- ❏ Pepcid
- ❏ Pepcid AC
- ❏ Peptavlon
- ❏ peptidase
- ❏ Pepto-Bismol
- ❏ Pepto-Bismol Max
- ❏ Pepto-Bismol InstaCool
- ❏ peptolide
- ❏ Perampanel
- ❏ Perbuterol
- ❏ Percocet
- ❏ Percodan
- ❏ Percogesic
- ❏ Percolone
- ❏ Perdiem
- ❏ Perflutren lipid microspheres
- ❏ Perform
- ❏ Perforomist
- ❏ pergolide
- ❏ Pergonal
- ❏ Periactin
- ❏ Peri-Colace
- ❏ Peridex
- ❏ Peridin-C
- ❏ perindopril erbumine
- ❏ Periochip
- ❏ Periogard
- ❏ Periostat
- ❏ Perlabella
- ❏ Perlane
- ❏ Permax
- ❏ permethrin
- ❏ perphenazine
- ❏ Persantine
- ❏ pethidine
- ❏ Pfizerpen
- ❏ Phazyme
- ❏ Phenaphen

- ❏ phenazopyridine
- ❏ Phencyclidine
- ❏ phendimetrazine tartrate
- ❏ phenelzine
- ❏ Phenergan
- ❏ pheniramine
- ❏ Phenobarbital
- ❏ phenol
- ❏ phenolphthalein
- ❏ phenothiazine
- ❏ phenoxybenzamine
- ❏ phenserine
- ❏ phentermine
- ❏ phentolamine
- ❏ phenurone
- ❏ phenylalanine
- ❏ phenylazo-diamino-pyridine
- ❏ phenylephrine
- ❏ phenylprine
- ❏ phenylpropanolamine
- ❏ phenyl salicylate
- ❏ phenyltoloxamine
- ❏ Phenytek
- ❏ phenytoin
- ❏ Phillips Milk of Magnesia
- ❏ pHisoDerm
- ❏ pHisoHex
- ❏ Phoschol
- ❏ PhosLo
- ❏ phosphatidylcholine
- ❏ phosphodiesterase inhibitor
- ❏ phospholine iodide
- ❏ phosphomycin
- ❏ Photofrin
- ❏ Phrenilin Forte
- ❏ Phyllocontin
- ❏ physostigmine
- ❏ phytoene

P

- ❏ phytoestrogen
- ❏ phytofluene
- ❏ phytonadione
- ❏ Phytoplex
- ❏ phytosterol blocker
- ❏ Phyto-Vite
- ❏ Picovir
- ❏ Pilocar
- ❏ pilocarpine
- ❏ Pilocel
- ❏ Pima
- ❏ pimecrolimus
- ❏ pimozide
- ❏ pindolol
- ❏ Pin-Rid
- ❏ pioglitazone
- ❏ Pipecuronium
- ❏ piperacillin
- ❏ Pipracil
- ❏ pirbuterol
- ❏ Pirfenidone
- ❏ piroxicam
- ❏ pitavastatin
- ❏ Pitocin
- ❏ Pitressin Synthetic
- ❏ pixantrone
- ❏ Pixuvri
- ❏ PKC
- ❏ Placidyl
- ❏ Plan B
- ❏ Plan B One-Step
- ❏ plantago ovata
- ❏ Plaquenil
- ❏ PLAS+SD
- ❏ Plasbumin
- ❏ Plasma-Lyte
- ❏ Plasmanate
- ❏ Plasma-Plex

P

- ❏ plasma protein fraction
- ❏ Plasmatein
- ❏ Platinol-AQ
- ❏ Plavix
- ❏ Pleconaril
- ❏ Plegisol
- ❏ Plenaxis
- ❏ Plendil
- ❏ plerixafor
- ❏ Pletal
- ❏ Plexion
- ❏ plicamycin
- ❏ PMS Theophylline
- ❏ PN 400
- ❏ pneumococcal 13-valent
- ❏ Pneumomist
- ❏ Pneumotussin HC
- ❏ Pneumovax
- ❏ Pnu-Imune 23
- ❏ Podocon
- ❏ podofilox
- ❏ podophyllin
- ❏ polidocanol
- ❏ polifeprosan
- ❏ polistirex
- ❏ Polocaine
- ❏ Polycitra
- ❏ polyethylene glycol
- ❏ Polygam S/D
- ❏ PolyHeme
- ❏ Polyhistine
- ❏ Polymox
- ❏ polymyxin
- ❏ polypeptide
- ❏ Polyphenon E
- ❏ polysaccharide iron
- ❏ Polyspectrin
- ❏ Polysporin

P

P

- ❑ Polytar shampoo
- ❑ polythiazide
- ❑ Polytrim
- ❑ polyurethane
- ❑ polyvinyl chloride
- ❑ Poly-Vi-Sol
- ❑ POMP
- ❑ Ponaris
- ❑ Pond's
- ❑ Ponstel
- ❑ Pontocaine
- ❑ Poractant Alfa
- ❑ porfimer sodium
- ❑ Portia
- ❑ posaconazole
- ❑ Posicor
- ❑ Potaba
- ❑ Potaba envules
- ❑ potassium bitartrate
- ❑ potassium chloride
- ❑ potassium citrate
- ❑ Potiga
- ❑ postassium sulfate
- ❑ povidone/iodine
- ❑ Pradaxa
- ❑ pralatrexate
- ❑ pralidoxime chloride
- ❑ Pramilet
- ❑ pramipexole
- ❑ pramlintide
- ❑ Pramosone
- ❑ pramoxine
- ❑ Pranactin
- ❑ PrandiMet
- ❑ Prandin
- ❑ prasugrel
- ❑ Pravachol
- ❑ Pravagard

- ❑ pravastatin
- ❑ pravastin
- ❑ Prax
- ❑ praziquantel
- ❑ prazosin
- ❑ PreCare Prenatal
- ❑ Precedex
- ❑ Precose
- ❑ Pred Forte
- ❑ prednicarbate
- ❑ Prednicen
- ❑ prednisolone
- ❑ prednisone
- ❑ Prefrin
- ❑ Pregabalin
- ❑ Pregnyl
- ❑ Prelay
- ❑ Prelone
- ❑ Prelu-2
- ❑ Premarin
- ❑ PremesissRX
- ❑ Premphase
- ❑ Prempro
- ❑ Premsyn
- ❑ Prenate Ultra
- ❑ Preparation H
- ❑ Prepcat
- ❑ Prepidil
- ❑ PreScrub
- ❑ Prestara
- ❑ Prevacid
- ❑ Prevalite
- ❑ Preven
- ❑ Prevident
- ❑ Prevnar
- ❑ Prevnar 13
- ❑ Prevpac
- ❑ Prezista

P

P

- ❏ prGCD
- ❏ Prialt
- ❏ Prid
- ❏ Priftin
- ❏ prilocaine
- ❏ Prilosec
- ❏ Prilosec OTC
- ❏ Primacare
- ❏ Primacor
- ❏ primaquine
- ❏ Primatene
- ❏ Primatene mist
- ❏ Primaxin
- ❏ primidone
- ❏ Primsol
- ❏ Principen
- ❏ Prinivil
- ❏ Prinzide
- ❏ Priscoline
- ❏ Pristiq
- ❏ Privigen
- ❏ ProAir HFA
- ❏ ProAmatine
- ❏ probenecid
- ❏ Probiata
- ❏ probiotics
- ❏ Probiotica
- ❏ Probucol
- ❏ procainamide
- ❏ ProcalAmine
- ❏ Procanbid
- ❏ procarbazine
- ❏ Procardia
- ❏ Prochieve
- ❏ prochlorperazine
- ❏ Procleix
- ❏ Pro Clearz
- ❏ ProClude

- ❏ Procosa II
- ❏ Procrit
- ❏ Proctocort
- ❏ Proctocream HC
- ❏ Proctofoam HC
- ❏ procyclidine
- ❏ Procylon
- ❏ Procytox
- ❏ Prodium
- ❏ Profasi
- ❏ Profen
- ❏ Profilnine SD
- ❏ Proflavanol
- ❏ Progesin
- ❏ Progestasert System
- ❏ progesterone
- ❏ Proglycem
- ❏ Prograf
- ❏ Prograniq
- ❏ proguanil
- ❏ ProHance
- ❏ ProHIBiT
- ❏ Prohim
- ❏ Prolab
- ❏ Prolastin
- ❏ Prolatis'
- ❏ Proleukin
- ❏ Prolex
- ❏ Prolia
- ❏ Prolixin
- ❏ Proloprim
- ❏ ProMACE-CytaBOM
- ❏ Promacta
- ❏ promazine
- ❏ Promensil
- ❏ Prometh
- ❏ promethazine
- ❏ Prometrium

P

- Pronestyl
- Pronto
- pronutra protein
- Propade
- propafenone
- Propagest
- propantheline
- Proparacaine
- propatyl nitrate
- Propecia
- Propel Implant
- Prophyllin CCC
- propicillin
- Propine C Cap
- propiolactone
- Proplex T
- propofol
- propoxyphene
- propoxyphene napsylate
- propranolol
- Propulsid
- propyl alcohol
- propylene glycol
- propylhexedrine
- propylthiouracil
- Proquad
- Proquin XR
- Prosacea
- Proscar
- Prosed
- ProSol
- ProSom
- prostaglandin
- Prostaphlin
- Prostata
- ProStep
- Prostigmin
- Prostin

P

- protamine sulfate
- protamine zinc
- protease
- protease inhibitor
- Protenate
- proteolytic enzyme
- Protex
- Protid
- protirelin
- proton pump inhibitor
- Protonix
- Protopam chloride
- Protophylline
- Protopic
- Protostat
- protriptyline
- Protropin
- Protuss
- ProVectin
- Provenge
- Proventil
- Provera
- Provigil
- Provocholine
- Proxacol
- ProXtreme
- Prozac
- Prudoxin
- Prunelax
- pseudoephedrine
- pseudoephedrine sulfate
- psoralens
- Psorcon
- Psoriasin gel
- psyllium
- PTK 787
- Pulexn DM
- Pumactant

P

- ❑ Pulmicort Flexhaler
- ❑ Pulmicort Respules
- ❑ Pulmicort Turbuhaler
- ❑ Pulmophylline
- ❑ Pulmozyme
- ❑ PureTrim
- ❑ Puricase
- ❑ Puri-Clens
- ❑ Purinethol
- ❑ Purpose
- ❑ Pylera
- ❑ Pylori-Chek
- ❑ pyrantel pamoate
- ❑ pyrazinamide
- ❑ Pyridium
- ❑ pyridostigmine
- ❑ pyridoxine
- ❑ pyrilamine
- ❑ pyrimethamine
- ❑ pyrithione

Q

- ❑ QAB149
- ❑ Q-Bid
- ❑ Qlaira
- ❑ Qnexa
- ❑ Quaalude
- ❑ quadazocine
- ❑ quadrivalent
- ❑ Quadramet
- ❑ Quadrinal
- ❑ Qualaquin
- ❑ Quanterra
- ❑ Quarzan
- ❑ Quasense
- ❑ Quelicin

Q

- ❑ Quenalin
- ❑ Questran
- ❑ quetiapine
- ❑ Quibron
- ❑ quinacrine
- ❑ Quinaglute
- ❑ quinalan
- ❑ quinalbarbitone
- ❑ quinaldine blue
- ❑ Quinamm
- ❑ quinapril
- ❑ quinethazone
- ❑ Quin-G
- ❑ Quinidex
- ❑ quinidine
- ❑ quinine
- ❑ quinolone
- ❑ Quin-Release
- ❑ Quintex
- ❑ quinupristin
- ❑ Quixin
- ❑ Qutenza
- ❑ QVAR

R

- ❑ RabAvert
- ❑ rabeprazole
- ❑ Racivir
- ❑ Radiance injection
- ❑ Radiesse
- ❑ Radiogardase
- ❑ Ralivia
- ❑ raloxifene
- ❑ raltegravir
- ❑ ramelteon
- ❑ ramipril

R	R

- Ranexa
- ranibizumab
- ranitidine
- ranolazine
- rapacuronium
- Rapaflo
- Rapamune
- Rapinex
- Rapinyl
- Raplon
- Raptiva
- rasagiline mesylate
- rasburicase
- Rasilez
- Rauwolfia serpentina
- Rauzide
- Raxar
- raxibacumab
- Rayataz
- Razadyne
- Reality
- Rebetol
- Rebetron
- Rebif
- Reclast
- Reclipsen
- Recombinant OspA
- Recombinate
- Recombivax
- Recothrom
- Rectiv
- Redox
- Refacto
- Refludan
- Refresh Celluvisc
- Refresh Liquigel
- Refresh Optive
- Refresh P.M.

- Refresh Tears
- regadenoson
- Regasporin
- Regitine
- Reglan
- Regonol
- Regranex
- Regroton
- Regulex
- Regutol
- Rehydralyte
- Reishimax
- Relafen
- Relagesic
- Releev
- Relenza
- Relistor
- Relpax
- Remeron
- REMERONSolTab
- Remicade
- remifentanil
- Reminyl
- Remodulin
- Remoxy
- Remune
- Remular
- Renacidin irrigation
- Renagel
- RenAmin
- Renax
- Renedil
- Renese
- Renografin 60
- Reno-M-30
- Renova
- Renovue
- ReNu

R	R

- ❑ Renvela
- ❑ ReoPro
- ❑ repaglinide
- ❑ RepHresh
- ❑ Replagal
- ❑ Replens
- ❑ Repronex
- ❑ Requip
- ❑ Rescinnamine
- ❑ Rescon
- ❑ Rescriptor
- ❑ Rescula
- ❑ reserpine
- ❑ resorcinol
- ❑ Respa A.R.M.
- ❑ Respa-DM
- ❑ Respa-GF
- ❑ Respahist
- ❑ Respaire-SR
- ❑ Respbid
- ❑ RESPeRATE
- ❑ RespiGam
- ❑ Respihaler
- ❑ Respinol
- ❑ Resporal
- ❑ Restanza
- ❑ Restasis
- ❑ Restoril
- ❑ Restylane
- ❑ retapamulin
- ❑ Retavase
- ❑ Reteplase
- ❑ Retigabine
- ❑ Retin-A
- ❑ Retisert
- ❑ Retrovir
- ❑ Revatio
- ❑ Reversol

- ❑ Revex
- ❑ ReVia
- ❑ Revitalift
- ❑ Revivexxx
- ❑ Revlimid
- ❑ Rexata
- ❑ Reyataz
- ❑ Rezira
- ❑ Rezulin
- ❑ R-Gene 10
- ❑ Rheomacrodex
- ❑ Rheumatrex
- ❑ Rhinocort Aqua
- ❑ Rhinogesic
- ❑ Rhinosyn-X
- ❑ RhoGam
- ❑ Rhophylac
- ❑ Rhucin
- ❑ Rhuli
- ❑ RhuMAb-E25
- ❑ RiaSTAP
- ❑ ribasphere
- ❑ ribavirin
- ❑ riboflavin
- ❑ ricinoleic acid
- ❑ Ricola
- ❑ ridaforolimus
- ❑ Ridaura
- ❑ Rid Mousse
- ❑ rifabutin
- ❑ Rifadin
- ❑ Rifamate
- ❑ rifampin
- ❑ rifapentine
- ❑ Rifater
- ❑ rifaximin
- ❑ rilonacept
- ❑ rilpivirine

R	R

- ❏ Rilutek
- ❏ riluzole
- ❏ Rimactane
- ❏ rimantadine
- ❏ rimonabant
- ❏ Rimso
- ❏ rinfabate
- ❏ Riomet
- ❏ Riopan
- ❏ Riquent
- ❏ risedronate
- ❏ Risperdal
- ❏ Risperdal Consta
- ❏ risperidone
- ❏ Ritalin
- ❏ Ritodrine
- ❏ ritonavir
- ❏ Rituxan
- ❏ rituximab
- ❏ rivaroxaban
- ❏ rivastigmine
- ❏ rizatriptan
- ❏ RMS suppository
- ❏ Robaxin
- ❏ Robaxisal
- ❏ Robinul
- ❏ Robitussin
- ❏ Robitussin CF
- ❏ Robitussin DAC
- ❏ Robitussin DM
- ❏ Robitussin DM Max
- ❏ Roc
- ❏ Rocaltrol
- ❏ Rocephin
- ❏ rocuronium bromide
- ❏ rofecoxib
- ❏ Roferon-A
- ❏ roflumilast

- ❏ Rogaine
- ❏ Rogitine
- ❏ Rohto Hydra
- ❏ Rohto V
- ❏ Rohto Zi
- ❏ Rohypnol
- ❏ Rolaids
- ❏ Rolaids softchews
- ❏ Romazicon
- ❏ romidepsin
- ❏ romiplostim
- ❏ Rondec
- ❏ roofie
- ❏ ropinirole
- ❏ ropivacaine
- ❏ Rosac wash
- ❏ Rose Bengal
- ❏ Risets strips
- ❏ rosiglitazone
- ❏ rosuvastatin
- ❏ Rotahaler
- ❏ Rotarix
- ❏ RotaShield
- ❏ Rotateq
- ❏ rotavirus
- ❏ rotigotine
- ❏ Rowasa enema
- ❏ ROX-888
- ❏ Roxanol
- ❏ Roxicet
- ❏ Roxicodone
- ❏ Roxilox
- ❏ Roxiprin
- ❏ Rozerem
- ❏ RSV-IGIV
- ❏ RU-486 [mifepristone]
- ❏ Rubex
- ❏ rufinamide

R

- ❑ Rufludan
- ❑ Rum-K
- ❑ Rutoside
- ❑ Ruxolitinib
- ❑ Ryna-12
- ❑ Rynatan
- ❑ Rynatuss
- ❑ Rythmol
- ❑ Rythmol SR
- ❑ Ryzolt

S

- ❑ Sabril
- ❑ sacosidase
- ❑ Safe 4 Hours
- ❑ Safe-Tussin
- ❑ Saflutan
- ❑ Safyral
- ❑ St. Ives
- ❑ St. John's Wort
- ❑ St. Joseph Aspirin
- ❑ Saizen
- ❑ SalAc
- ❑ Sal-Acid plaster
- ❑ Salactic film
- ❑ Salagen
- ❑ Salflex
- ❑ salicylamide
- ❑ salicylic acid
- ❑ salicylsalicylic acid
- ❑ salmeterol xinafoate
- ❑ Salonpas
- ❑ Salonsip Aqua Patch
- ❑ Sal-Plant gel
- ❑ salsalate
- ❑ Saluron

S

- ❑ Salutensin
- ❑ SAM-e
- ❑ Sambucol
- ❑ Samsca
- ❑ Sanctura
- ❑ Sanctura XR
- ❑ Sancuso
- ❑ Sandimmune
- ❑ Sandoglobulin
- ❑ Sandostatin
- ❑ SangCya
- ❑ Sanorex
- ❑ Sansert
- ❑ Santyl
- ❑ Saphris
- ❑ sapropterin dihydrochloride
- ❑ saquinavir
- ❑ Sarafem
- ❑ Sarapin
- ❑ sargramostim
- ❑ Sarna
- ❑ Sativex
- ❑ Satogesic
- ❑ Savella
- ❑ Saw Palmetto
- ❑ saxagliptin
- ❑ SBR-Lipocream
- ❑ S-Caine Peel
- ❑ Scalpicin
- ❑ Scar Away
- ❑ Scarguard
- ❑ SCE-A
- ❑ Schick
- ❑ Scleromate
- ❑ Sclerosol intrapleural
- ❑ scopolamine
- ❑ scopolamine hydrobromide
- ❑ Sculptra

S

- ❏ Sea-Band
- ❏ Sea-Clens
- ❏ Seasonale
- ❏ Seasonique
- ❏ Sebazole
- ❏ Sebulex
- ❏ secobarbital
- ❏ Seconal
- ❏ SecreFlo
- ❏ Secretin
- ❏ Sectral
- ❏ Sedapap
- ❏ selegiline
- ❏ selenium
- ❏ selenium sulfide
- ❏ selenomethionine
- ❏ Selsun
- ❏ Selzentry
- ❏ Semicid
- ❏ Semilente
- ❏ Semprex
- ❏ Sen Lo Fen
- ❏ senna
- ❏ sennosides
- ❏ Sen-Sei-Ro
- ❏ Senokot
- ❏ Senokot-S
- ❏ SenokotXTRA
- ❏ Sensipar
- ❏ Sensorcaine
- ❏ Sepracor
- ❏ Septocaine
- ❏ Septra
- ❏ Ser-Ap-Es
- ❏ Serax
- ❏ Serdolect
- ❏ Serentil
- ❏ Serevent

S

- ❏ sermorelin
- ❏ Seromycin
- ❏ Serophene
- ❏ Seroquel
- ❏ Seroquel XR
- ❏ Serostim
- ❏ serotonin uptake inhibitor
- ❏ SERPACWA
- ❏ sertaconazole
- ❏ sertindole
- ❏ sertraline
- ❏ serum albumin
- ❏ Serutan
- ❏ Serzone
- ❏ sevelamer
- ❏ sevoflurane
- ❏ Sexativa Plus
- ❏ Sexelle
- ❏ shea butter
- ❏ shikonin
- ❏ Sibilium
- ❏ sibutramine
- ❏ sildenafil citrate
- ❏ Silenor
- ❏ Silmycin
- ❏ silodosin
- ❏ Silvadene
- ❏ silver nitrate
- ❏ silver protein, mild
- ❏ silver sulfadiazine
- ❏ Simcor
- ❏ simethicone
- ❏ Similasan
- ❏ Simply Sleep
- ❏ Simponi
- ❏ Simulect
- ❏ simvastatin
- ❏ Sinarest

S

- ❏ Sincalide
- ❏ Sine-Aid
- ❏ Sinemet
- ❏ Sine-Off
- ❏ Sinequan
- ❏ Sine-Relief
- ❏ Sinex
- ❏ Singulair
- ❏ SinoFresh
- ❏ Sinografin
- ❏ SinuCleanse
- ❏ Sinulin
- ❏ Sinumist
- ❏ Sinutab
- ❏ Sinutuss
- ❏ Sinuvent
- ❏ sipuleucel-T
- ❏ sirolimus
- ❏ sitagliptin
- ❏ Skelaxin
- ❏ Skelid
- ❏ Skintimate
- ❏ Sleep-Eze
- ❏ Sleep-Eze-3
- ❏ Sleep-Eze D
- ❏ Sleepinal
- ❏ Sleep-Max PM
- ❏ Sloan's liniment
- ❏ Slo-Bid
- ❏ Slo-Fe
- ❏ Slo-Niacin
- ❏ Slo-Phyllin
- ❏ Slow-Mag
- ❏ SnoreStop
- ❏ SNO Strips
- ❏ sodium acid phosphate
- ❏ sodium benzoate
- ❏ sodium bicarbonate

S

- ❏ sodium brevital
- ❏ sodium chloride
- ❏ sodium citrate
- ❏ sodium diphosphate
- ❏ sodium ferric gluconate
- ❏ sodium fluoride
- ❏ sodium hyaluronate
- ❏ sodium oxybate
- ❏ sodium oxychlorosene
- ❏ sodium pentothal
- ❏ sodium phenylacetate
- ❏ sodium phosphate
- ❏ sodium propionate
- ❏ sodium sulamyd
- ❏ sodium sulfacetamide
- ❏ sodium sulfate
- ❏ Sojourn Sevoflurane
- ❏ Solage
- ❏ Solaquin
- ❏ Solaraze
- ❏ Solarcaine
- ❏ Solbar
- ❏ Solganal
- ❏ solifenacin succinate
- ❏ Soliris
- ❏ Solodyn
- ❏ Solo Slim
- ❏ Soltamox
- ❏ Solu-Cortef
- ❏ Solu-Medrol
- ❏ Solu-Phyllin
- ❏ Solurex
- ❏ Solzira
- ❏ Soma Compound
- ❏ SomatoKine
- ❏ somatostatin
- ❏ somatrem
- ❏ somatropin

S	**S**

❑ Somatuline Autogel
❑ Somatuline Depot
❑ Somavert
❑ Sominex
❑ Sonata
❑ SonoRX
❑ Soothe XP
❑ sorafenib
❑ sorbitol
❑ Sorbitrate
❑ Soriatane
❑ Sorilux
❑ Sorine
❑ sotalol
❑ Sotradecol
❑ Sotret
❑ soy oil
❑ Spacer
❑ sparfloxacin
❑ SparVax
❑ Spectazole
❑ Spectracef
❑ Spectrobid
❑ Spenco 2nd Skin Scar
❑ spinosad
❑ spironolactone
❑ spiramycin
❑ Spiriva
❑ Spiriva HandiHaler
❑ Sporanox
❑ Sportscreme
❑ Sprintek
❑ Sprix
❑ Sprycel
❑ Sronyx
❑ SSD cream
❑ SSD AF cream
❑ SSKI solution

❑ Staccato
❑ Stacker 2
❑ Stadol NS
❑ Stalevo
❑ Staminex
❑ Stanback
❑ stanozolol
❑ StaphAseptic
❑ Starlix
❑ Staticin
❑ Statrol
❑ stavudine
❑ Stavzor
❑ Staxyn
❑ Stedesa
❑ Stelara
❑ Stelazine
❑ Sterapred
❑ SteriLid
❑ Stilbestrol
❑ stilphostrol
❑ Stopain
❑ Stoxil
❑ Strattera
❑ Streptase
❑ streptokinase
❑ Streptomycin
❑ streptozocin
❑ Striant
❑ Stridex
❑ StriVectin-HS
❑ StriVectin-SD
❑ Stromectol
❑ Strovite
❑ Stye
❑ SU-101
❑ SU 11248
❑ Sublimaze

S	S

- Sublinox
- Suboxone
- Subutex
- succimer
- succinylcholine
- succuss cineraria maritma
- Sucraid
- sucralfate
- Sucrets
- Sudafed
- Sudafed OM
- Sufenta
- Sufentanil
- Sugen
- Sulamyd
- Sular
- sulbactam sodium
- sulfabenzamide
- Sulfacet
- sulfacetamide sodium
- sulfadiazine
- sulfadoxine
- sulfamerazine
- sulfamethiazine
- sulfamethizole
- sulfamethoxazole
- Sulfamide
- Sulfamylon cream
- sulfanilamide
- SulfaPred
- sulfasalazine
- sulfinpyrazone
- sulfisoxazole
- sulfonamide
- Sulfonylurea
- Sulfoxyl
- sulfur
- sulindac

- Sultrin
- sumatriptan
- Sumavel DosePro
- Summer's Eve
- Sumycin
- sunitinib
- Sunril
- Supartz
- Super EPA
- Superfak
- superoxide dismutase
- Supprelin
- Supprelin LA
- Suprane
- Suprax
- Suprefact
- Suprep
- Sure Sleep
- Surfak
- Surfaxin
- Surgidine
- Surgilube
- Surmontil
- Survanta
- Sus-Phrine
- Sustaire
- Sustenex
- Sustiva
- Sutent
- Swabplus
- Swiss Kriss
- Sylatron
- Syllact
- Symadine
- Symbicort
- Symbyax
- Symiotropin
- Symlin

S

- ❏ Symmetrel
- ❏ Symphasic
- ❏ Synagis
- ❏ Synalar
- ❏ Synalgos-DC
- ❏ Synarel
- ❏ Synemol
- ❏ Synera
- ❏ Synercid
- ❏ SynergyDefense
- ❏ Synophylate
- ❏ Synphasic
- ❏ Syprine
- ❏ Syn-Rx
- ❏ Synthroid
- ❏ Syntocinon
- ❏ Synvisc
- ❏ Synvisc-One
- ❏ Synovium
- ❏ Syprine
- ❏ SYR-322
- ❏ Systane

T

- ❏ Tabloid
- ❏ TAC-3
- ❏ Taclonex
- ❏ tacrine
- ❏ tacrolimus
- ❏ tadalafil
- ❏ Tafamidis
- ❏ tafluprost
- ❏ Tagamet
- ❏ Talacen
- ❏ taliglucerase alfa
- ❏ Talwin

T

- ❏ Tambocor
- ❏ Tamiflu
- ❏ tamoxifen
- ❏ tamsulosin
- ❏ Tanac
- ❏ Tanafed
- ❏ Tandem
- ❏ TAO
- ❏ Tapazole
- ❏ tapentadol
- ❏ Tarceva
- ❏ Targretin
- ❏ Tarka
- ❏ Tasigna
- ❏ Tasmar
- ❏ Taurine
- ❏ Tavist D
- ❏ Taxol
- ❏ Taxotere
- ❏ tazarotene
- ❏ Tazicef
- ❏ Tazidime
- ❏ tazobactam
- ❏ Tazorac
- ❏ Taztia
- ❏ TC7 [Interceed]
- ❏ TE Anatoxal Berna
- ❏ Teagreen
- ❏ Tears Naturale
- ❏ Tecnu
- ❏ Teczem
- ❏ Teflaro
- ❏ tegaserod maleate
- ❏ Tegretol
- ❏ Tegison
- ❏ Tegopen
- ❏ Tegreen 97
- ❏ Tekamlo

T

- ❏ Tekturna
- ❏ Tekturna HCT
- ❏ telaprevir
- ❏ telavancin
- ❏ Telbermin
- ❏ telbivudine
- ❏ Tel-E-Dose products
- ❏ Tel-E-Ject products
- ❏ Telepaque
- ❏ telithromycin
- ❏ telmesteine
- ❏ telmisartan
- ❏ Temaril
- ❏ temazepam
- ❏ Temodar
- ❏ Temovate
- ❏ temozolomide
- ❏ temsirolimus
- ❏ Tencon
- ❏ tenecteplase
- ❏ Tenex
- ❏ teniposide
- ❏ tenofovir disoproxil fumarate
- ❏ Tenoretic
- ❏ Tenormin
- ❏ Tensilon
- ❏ Tenuate
- ❏ Tequin
- ❏ Terazol
- ❏ terazosin
- ❏ terbinafine
- ❏ terbutaline
- ❏ terconazole
- ❏ Teril
- ❏ teriparatide
- ❏ terlipressin
- ❏ terpin hydrate
- ❏ Terra-Cortril

T

- ❏ Terramycin
- ❏ tesamorelin
- ❏ Teslac
- ❏ Teslascan
- ❏ TESPA [TSPA]
- ❏ Tessalon
- ❏ Tessalon Perles
- ❏ Testerex
- ❏ Testim
- ❏ Testoderm TTS
- ❏ testolactone
- ❏ Testopel Pellet
- ❏ testosterone
- ❏ testosterone cypionate
- ❏ testosterone enanthate
- ❏ Testred
- ❏ tetrabenazine
- ❏ tetracaine
- ❏ tetracycline
- ❏ tetrahydrozoline
- ❏ Tetramune
- ❏ Tetrazene ES-50
- ❏ Teveten
- ❏ Teveten HCT
- ❏ Tev-Tropin
- ❏ Thalidomide
- ❏ Thalitone
- ❏ Thalomid
- ❏ thallus chloride
- ❏ Tham
- ❏ Theo-24
- ❏ Theo-250
- ❏ Theo-Bid
- ❏ Theochron
- ❏ Theoclear
- ❏ Theocot
- ❏ Theo-dur
- ❏ Theolair

T

- Theomer
- theophylline
- theophylline anydrous
- Theostat
- Thiotepa
- Theo-Time
- Theovent
- Theo-X
- TheraCys
- Theradent
- TheraFlu
- Thera-Gesic
- Theramycin
- TheraPatch
- TheraTears
- ThermaCare
- Thermage
- ThermoDox
- Thermogenics
- thiabendazole
- thiamine
- thiamine disulfide
- thiazolidinedione
- thiethylperazine
- Thimerosal
- Thin-Patch
- ThinPrep
- Thinz
- thioguanine
- Thiola
- thiobarbiturates
- thiobutabarbital
- thiopental sodium
- Thioplex
- thioridazine
- thiotepa
- thiothixene
- Thonzonium

T

- Thorazine
- Thrombate III
- Thrombin-JMI
- Thylline
- Thymoglobulin
- Thymol
- thymus polypeptide
- Thyrel TRH
- Thyrogen
- thyroid
- Thyrolar
- ThyroSafe
- ThyroShield
- ThyroStart
- Thyro-Tab
- Thyrotropin Alfa
- tiagabine
- Tiazac
- Tibolone
- ticagrelor
- Ticar
- ticarcillin
- TICE BCG
- Ticlid
- ticlopidine
- Tifacogin
- Tigan
- tigecycline
- Tiger Balm
- Tikosyn
- Tilade Inhaler
- Tilia FE
- tiludronate
- Timentin
- TimeOut
- Timolide
- timolol
- Timoptic

| T | T |

- ❏ Timoptic-XE
- ❏ Tinactin
- ❏ Tinamed
- ❏ Tindamax
- ❏ Tine test PPD
- ❏ Tineacide
- ❏ tinidazole
- ❏ tinzaparin
- ❏ tioconazole
- ❏ tiopronin
- ❏ tiotropium bromide
- ❏ tipranavir
- ❏ Tirofiban
- ❏ Tisseel [Fibrin Sealant]
- ❏ Titralac
- ❏ tizanidine
- ❏ TMC278
- ❏ TNKase
- ❏ TOBI
- ❏ Tobradex
- ❏ tobramycin
- ❏ Tobrex
- ❏ tocainide
- ❏ tocilizumab
- ❏ tocopheryl acetate
- ❏ Tofipan
- ❏ Tofipan-Z
- ❏ Tofranil
- ❏ Tolamide
- ❏ tolazamide
- ❏ tolazoline
- ❏ tolbutamide
- ❏ tolcapone
- ❏ Tolectin
- ❏ Tolinase
- ❏ tolmetin sodium
- ❏ tolnaftate
- ❏ tolterodine

- ❏ tolvaptan
- ❏ Tomocat
- ❏ Tonocard
- ❏ Tonopaque
- ❏ Topamax
- ❏ Topicort
- ❏ topiramate
- ❏ topotecan
- ❏ Topricin
- ❏ Toprol XL
- ❏ Toradol
- ❏ torcetrapib
- ❏ Torecan
- ❏ toremifene
- ❏ Torisel
- ❏ Tornalate
- ❏ torsemide
- ❏ tositumomab
- ❏ Totect
- ❏ Totephan crème
- ❏ Toviaz
- ❏ TPA
- ❏ TPN electrolytes
- ❏ Trabectedin
- ❏ Tracleer
- ❏ Tracrium
- ❏ Tradjenta
- ❏ Tramadol
- ❏ tranadik
- ❏ Trancopal
- ❏ Trandate
- ❏ trandolapril
- ❏ Transderm-Nitro patch
- ❏ Transderm SCOP patch
- ❏ Tranex
- ❏ tranexamic acid
- ❏ Tranxene
- ❏ trastuzumab

T	T

- ❑ Trasylol
- ❑ Traumeel
- ❑ Travasol
- ❑ Travatan Z
- ❑ Travoprost
- ❑ trazodone
- ❑ Treanda
- ❑ Trecator-SC
- ❑ Trelstar
- ❑ Trelstar LA
- ❑ Trental
- ❑ treprostinil
- ❑ tretinoin
- ❑ Trexall
- ❑ Trexan
- ❑ Trexima
- ❑ Treximet
- ❑ Triactin
- ❑ triamcinolone
- ❑ Triam/HCTZ
- ❑ Triaminic
- ❑ Triaminic Softchews
- ❑ Triaminicin
- ❑ triamterene
- ❑ Tri-Sprintec
- ❑ Triavil
- ❑ Triaz
- ❑ triazolam
- ❑ Tribenzor
- ❑ tricarbocyanine
- ❑ trichlormethiazide
- ❑ tricitrates
- ❑ tricitrates SF
- ❑ TriCor
- ❑ TriDerma
- ❑ Tridesilon
- ❑ Tridil
- ❑ trientine

- ❑ Triesence
- ❑ trifluoperazine
- ❑ Trifluoper HCL
- ❑ trifluorothymidine
- ❑ trifluridine
- ❑ Triglide
- ❑ trihexyphenidyl
- ❑ TriHIBit
- ❑ Trikof-D
- ❑ Trilafon
- ❑ Trileptal
- ❑ Tri-Levlen
- ❑ Trilipix
- ❑ Trilisate
- ❑ Trilostane
- ❑ Tri-Luma Cream
- ❑ trimethobenzamide
- ❑ Trimethoprim
- ❑ trimetrexate
- ❑ trimipramine
- ❑ Trimox
- ❑ Trimpex
- ❑ Trinalin
- ❑ TriNessa
- ❑ Tri-Nasal
- ❑ Tri-Norinyl
- ❑ Trinsicon
- ❑ Triostat
- ❑ Tripedia
- ❑ Tripelennamine
- ❑ Triphasil
- ❑ triprolidine
- ❑ Triptans
- ❑ triptorelin pamoate
- ❑ Trisenox
- ❑ Trisoralen
- ❑ Tritec
- ❑ Tri-Thalmic

T

- ❏ Trivaris
- ❏ Trivora
- ❏ trivagizole
- ❏ Trizivir
- ❏ Trobicin
- ❏ troglitazone
- ❏ troleandomycin
- ❏ tromethamine
- ❏ Tronolane
- ❏ TrophAmine
- ❏ tropicacyl
- ❏ tropicamide
- ❏ trospium
- ❏ trospium chloride
- ❏ trovafloxacin
- ❏ Trovan
- ❏ Truphylline
- ❏ Trusopt
- ❏ Truvada
- ❏ Truxophylline
- ❏ Trypsin
- ❏ tryptophan
- ❏ Trysol
- ❏ TSPA
- ❏ T-Stat
- ❏ Tubersol
- ❏ Tucks
- ❏ Tums
- ❏ Tussafed
- ❏ Tussend
- ❏ Tussin
- ❏ Tussionex Pennkinetic
- ❏ Tussi-Organidin
- ❏ Tussizone
- ❏ TVP-1012
- ❏ Twinlab GTB Chromium
- ❏ Twinject
- ❏ Twinrix

T

- ❏ Twynsta
- ❏ Tygacil
- ❏ Tykerb
- ❏ Tylenol
- ❏ Tylenol caplets
- ❏ Tylenol geltabs
- ❏ Tylox
- ❏ Tyloxapol
- ❏ Tympagesic
- ❏ Typhim Vi
- ❏ tyrothrycin
- ❏ Tysabri
- ❏ Tyvaso
- ❏ Tyzeka

U

- ❏ U-90152S
- ❏ UK-68-798
- ❏ UK 92480
- ❏ Ulcine
- ❏ Ulesfia
- ❏ ulipristal acetate
- ❏ Uloric
- ❏ Ultane
- ❏ Ultiva
- ❏ Ultrabrom
- ❏ ULTRACEPT
- ❏ Ultracet
- ❏ Ultra-Fiber
- ❏ Ultralente
- ❏ Ultram
- ❏ Ultrase
- ❏ Ultra-TechneKow DTE
- ❏ Ultravate
- ❏ Ultravist
- ❏ Ultrazyme

U

- ❏ Unasyn
- ❏ undecylenic acid
- ❏ Undelenic
- ❏ Unguentine
- ❏ Unicap
- ❏ Unicontin
- ❏ Unidor
- ❏ Unifiber
- ❏ Unipen
- ❏ Uniphyl
- ❏ Uniretic
- ❏ Uniserts
- ❏ Unisol 4
- ❏ Unisom
- ❏ Unisyn
- ❏ Unithroid
- ❏ Uni-Tussin
- ❏ Univasc
- ❏ unoprostone
- ❏ Uprima
- ❏ Uracil
- ❏ urea
- ❏ Ureacin
- ❏ Ureaphil
- ❏ Urecholine
- ❏ Urex
- ❏ Uricalm
- ❏ Uridon
- ❏ Urimax
- ❏ Urised
- ❏ Urispas
- ❏ Uristat
- ❏ Urobak
- ❏ Urobiotic 250
- ❏ Urocit-K
- ❏ Urodine
- ❏ Urodol
- ❏ urofollitropin

U

- ❏ Urogesic
- ❏ Urokinase
- ❏ Uro-KP-Neutral
- ❏ Urolene blue
- ❏ Uro-Mag
- ❏ Uroplus
- ❏ Uroquid-Acid
- ❏ Urotrol
- ❏ Urovist Cysto
- ❏ UroXatral
- ❏ Urozide
- ❏ Ursinus
- ❏ Urso
- ❏ ursodeoxycholic acid
- ❏ Ursodiol
- ❏ Urso Forte
- ❏ ustekinumab
- ❏ Uvadex

V

- ❏ Vaccinia
- ❏ Vacuette
- ❏ Vagifem
- ❏ Vagisil
- ❏ Vagistat
- ❏ valacyclovir
- ❏ Valadol
- ❏ Valcyte
- ❏ valdecoxib
- ❏ Valergen
- ❏ Valerian
- ❏ valganciclovir
- ❏ Valisone
- ❏ Valium
- ❏ valproate sodium
- ❏ valproic acid

V

- Valrelease
- valrubicin
- valsartan
- Valstar
- Valtrex
- Valturna
- Vamate
- Vancenase
- Vanceril
- Vancocin
- Vancoled
- vancomycin
- vandetanib
- Vanex
- Vanicream
- Vaniqa
- Vanlev
- Vanos
- Vanoxide
- Vanquish
- Vantas
- Vantin
- VapoInhaler
- VapRub
- VapoSpray
- VapoSteam
- VapoSyrup
- VaporPatch
- Vaprisol
- VAQTA
- vardenafil
- varenicline
- Varidox
- Varivax
- VasClip
- Vascor
- Vascoray
- Vaseretic

V

- Vaseline
- Vasocidin
- VasoClear
- Vasocon
- Vasodilan
- Vaso-Lene
- Vasomax
- Vasoplex
- Vasopressin
- Vasosulf
- Vasotec
- Vasovist
- Vasoxyl
- Vatronol
- VCF Film
- Vectibix
- Vectical
- vecuronium
- Veet
- Veetids
- Velac
- velaglucerase alfa
- Velban
- Velcade
- Velosef
- Velosulin BR
- Velsar
- Veltin
- vemurafenib
- Venastat
- venlafaxine
- Venofer
- Venoglobulin-S
- Ventavis
- Ventolin
- Ventolin HFA
- VePesid
- Veramyst

V

- ❏ Verapamil
- ❏ Verdeso
- ❏ Veregen
- ❏ Verelan
- ❏ Vermox
- ❏ vernakalant
- ❏ Verrex
- ❏ Verrusol
- ❏ Versacaps
- ❏ Versed
- ❏ Versiclear
- ❏ verteporfin
- ❏ Vertigoheel
- ❏ Vesanoid
- ❏ VESIcare
- ❏ Vexol
- ❏ VFEND
- ❏ Viactiv
- ❏ Viadur
- ❏ Viagra
- ❏ VIAject
- ❏ Vibativ
- ❏ Vibramycin
- ❏ Vibra-Tabs
- ❏ Vicks
- ❏ Vicks 44D
- ❏ Vicks 44E
- ❏ Vicks Casero
- ❏ Vicks DayQuil
- ❏ Vicks Nyquil
- ❏ Vicks Sinex
- ❏ Vicks VapoRub
- ❏ Vicks VapoSteam
- ❏ Vicodin
- ❏ Vicon Forte
- ❏ Vicoprofen
- ❏ Victoza
- ❏ Victrelis

V

- ❏ vidarabine
- ❏ Vi-Daylin ADC
- ❏ Vidaza
- ❏ Videx
- ❏ vigabatrin
- ❏ Vigamox
- ❏ Viibryd
- ❏ vilazodone
- ❏ Vimovo
- ❏ Vimpat
- ❏ Vinarol
- ❏ vinblastine
- ❏ vincristine
- ❏ vindesine
- ❏ vinorelbine
- ❏ vinpocetine
- ❏ Viokase
- ❏ Vioxx
- ❏ Vira-A
- ❏ Viracept
- ❏ Viramune
- ❏ Virazole
- ❏ Viread
- ❏ Virilon
- ❏ Viroptic
- ❏ ViroSeq HIV-1
- ❏ Visculose
- ❏ viscum album
- ❏ Visicol
- ❏ Visine
- ❏ Visine-A
- ❏ Visine A.C.
- ❏ Visine L.R.
- ❏ Visine Tears
- ❏ Visipaque
- ❏ Visken
- ❏ Vismodegib
- ❏ Vistaril

V

❑ Vistide
❑ Visudyne Photodynamic
❑ VISUtein
❑ VISX
❑ Vitafol
❑ Vita-Minz
❑ Vitamist
❑ ViTelle Lurline PMS
❑ vitex agnus-castus
❑ Vitrase
❑ Vitrasert
❑ Vitravene
❑ Vivactil
❑ Viva-Drops
❑ Vivaglobin
❑ Vivarin
❑ Vivelle
❑ Vivelle-DOT
❑ Vivitrex
❑ Vivitrol
❑ Vivotif Berna
❑ VLB
❑ VM-26
❑ voclosporin
❑ Volmax
❑ Voltaren
❑ Vontrol
❑ Voriconazole
❑ vorinostat
❑ VoSol
❑ Votrient
❑ VP-16
❑ VPRIV
❑ Vumon
❑ Vytone
❑ Vytorin
❑ Vyvanse
❑ VZIG

W

❑ Wake-Up
❑ warfarin
❑ Wartner
❑ Wart-Off
❑ Water-Jel
❑ WC 3016
❑ WE Allergy
❑ Welchol
❑ Wellbutrin
❑ Westcort
❑ Wellcovorin
❑ West-Decon
❑ Westhroid
❑ Westrim
❑ Wigraine
❑ Wilate
❑ WinGel
❑ Winrgy
❑ WinRho SDF
❑ Winstrol
❑ witch hazel
❑ Wobenzym
❑ Wondra
❑ Woun'dres
❑ Wycillin
❑ Wydase
❑ Wygesic
❑ Wymox
❑ Wytensin

X

❑ Xalatan
❑ Xalkori
❑ Xanax
❑ xanthine oxidase inhibitor
❑ Xarelto
❑ Xcytrin

X

- ❑ Xeloda
- ❑ Xenaderm
- ❑ Xenadrine
- ❑ Xenazine
- ❑ Xenical
- ❑ Xeomin
- ❑ Xerac AC
- ❑ Xero-Lube
- ❑ Xgeva
- ❑ Xiaflex
- ❑ XiDay
- ❑ Xibrom
- ❑ Xience
- ❑ Xifaxan
- ❑ Xigris
- ❑ ximelagatran
- ❑ XL-3
- ❑ XM02
- ❑ Xolair
- ❑ Xolegel
- ❑ Xopenex
- ❑ XP13512
- ❑ X-Prep
- ❑ X-Seb T Plus
- ❑ XtremeLean
- ❑ X-Trozine
- ❑ Xylocaine
- ❑ Xylocard
- ❑ Xylometazoline
- ❑ Xyntha
- ❑ Xyrem
- ❑ Xyzal

Y

- ❑ Yaz
- ❑ Yasmin
- ❑ Yervoy

Y

- ❑ Yes to Carrots
- ❑ Yes to Cucumbers
- ❑ Yes to Tomatoes
- ❑ YF-VAX
- ❑ YM178
- ❑ Yocon
- ❑ Yodoxin
- ❑ Yohimar
- ❑ Yohimbe
- ❑ yohimbine
- ❑ Yohimex
- ❑ Youthgenes spray
- ❑ Yutopar

Z

- ❑ Zactima
- ❑ Zadaxin
- ❑ Zaditor
- ❑ zafirlukast
- ❑ Zagam
- ❑ Zalbin
- ❑ zalcitabine
- ❑ Zaleplon
- ❑ Zanaflex
- ❑ Zanamivar
- ❑ Zanfel
- ❑ Zanosar
- ❑ Zantac
- ❑ Zantrex
- ❑ Zantryl
- ❑ Zapex
- ❑ ZAPZYT
- ❑ Zarontin
- ❑ Zaroxolyn
- ❑ Zavesca
- ❑ Zeasorb
- ❑ zeaxanthin

Z

- ❏ Zebeta
- ❏ Zebrax
- ❏ Zebutal
- ❏ Zeel
- ❏ Zefazone
- ❏ Zegerid
- ❏ Zegerid OTC
- ❏ Zelapar
- ❏ Zelboraf
- ❏ Zelnorm
- ❏ Zelrix
- ❏ Zemaira
- ❏ Zemplar
- ❏ Zemuron
- ❏ Zenapax
- ❏ ZenChent
- ❏ Zenpep
- ❏ Zentase
- ❏ Zentrip
- ❏ Zenvia
- ❏ Zephrex
- ❏ Zerit
- ❏ Zeroxin
- ❏ Zestoretic
- ❏ Zestril
- ❏ Zetajet
- ❏ Zetar
- ❏ Zetia
- ❏ Zetran
- ❏ Zevalin
- ❏ Ziac
- ❏ Ziagen
- ❏ Ziana
- ❏ Zicam
- ❏ zidovudine
- ❏ Zilactin
- ❏ zileuton
- ❏ Zinacef

Z

- ❏ zinc
- ❏ zinc bisglycinate
- ❏ Zincon
- ❏ zinc oxide
- ❏ zinc pyrithione
- ❏ zinc sulfate
- ❏ Zincfrin
- ❏ Zinecard
- ❏ Zingo
- ❏ ziprasidone mesylate
- ❏ Zipsor
- ❏ Zirgan
- ❏ Zithromax
- ❏ Zithromax Z-Pak
- ❏ Zmax
- ❏ Zocor
- ❏ Zofran
- ❏ Zoladex
- ❏ zoledronate
- ❏ zoledronic acid
- ❏ Zolinza
- ❏ Zometa
- ❏ Zolmitriptan
- ❏ Zoloft
- ❏ zolpidem
- ❏ Zolpimist
- ❏ Zolyse
- ❏ Zometa
- ❏ Zomig
- ❏ Zomig-ZMT
- ❏ Zonalon
- ❏ Zonegran
- ❏ zonisamide
- ❏ Zorbtive
- ❏ Zorprin
- ❏ Zortress
- ❏ Zostavax
- ❏ zoster

Z

- ❑ Zosyn
- ❑ Zotarolimus
- ❑ zotepine
- ❑ Zoto-HC eardrops
- ❑ Zotrim
- ❑ Zotrix
- ❑ Zovia
- ❑ Zovirax
- ❑ Zuplenz
- ❑ Zutripro
- ❑ Zyban
- ❑ Zyclara
- ❑ Zydone
- ❑ Zyflo

Z

- ❑ Zyflo CR
- ❑ Zytiga
- ❑ Zylet
- ❑ Zyloprim
- ❑ ZymaDerm
- ❑ Zymar
- ❑ Zymase
- ❑ Zymenol
- ❑ Zyprexa
- ❑ Zyprexa Relprevv
- ❑ Zyrtec
- ❑ Zyrtec-D
- ❑ Zyvox

AIDS

- ❑ abacavir
- ❑ Agenerase
- ❑ AGT 088
- ❑ Aidsvax
- ❑ alitretinoin
- ❑ AmBisome
- ❑ AMD-070
- ❑ Amdoxovir
- ❑ Ampligen
- ❑ amprenavir
- ❑ Ao-Zidovudine
- ❑ Aptivus
- ❑ Aralen
- ❑ atazanavir
- ❑ atovaquone
- ❑ Atripla
- ❑ AVX101
- ❑ AZT
- ❑ azidothymidine
- ❑ Bactrim
- ❑ Biaxin
- ❑ Biozole
- ❑ CCR5 blockade
- ❑ CCR5 inhibitors
- ❑ cidofovir
- ❑ cobicistat
- ❑ Combivir
- ❑ Complera
- ❑ co-trimoxazole
- ❑ Crixivan
- ❑ cyanocobalamin
- ❑ Cytovene
- ❑ d4t
- ❑ DAPD
- ❑ Dapsone
- ❑ Daraprim
- ❑ darunavir
- ❑ daunorubicin

AIDS

- ❑ DaunoXome
- ❑ ddC
- ❑ delavirdine
- ❑ didanosine
- ❑ Diflucan
- ❑ Doxil
- ❑ Drabinol
- ❑ Edurant
- ❑ efavirenz
- ❑ Egrifta
- ❑ elvitegravir
- ❑ emtricitabine
- ❑ Emtriva
- ❑ ENF (T-20)
- ❑ Enfuvirtide
- ❑ Epivir
- ❑ Epzicom
- ❑ ethionamide
- ❑ etravirine
- ❑ Famvir
- ❑ Flumadine
- ❑ Formivirsen
- ❑ Fortovase
- ❑ Fosamprenavir
- ❑ foscarnete
- ❑ Foscavir
- ❑ fusion inhibitors
- ❑ Fuzeon
- ❑ ganciclovir
- ❑ HPA-23
- ❑ Hivid
- ❑ indinavir
- ❑ Infergen
- ❑ Integrase inhibitors
- ❑ Intelence
- ❑ interferon alfacon-1
- ❑ interferon alfa-N3
- ❑ Intron A

AIDS

AIDS

- Invirase
- Isentress
- Kaletra
- lamivudine
- Lexiva
- lopinavir
- Loramyc
- maraviroc
- Marinol
- Megace
- megestrol
- Mepron
- methylprednisolone
- miconazole
- miconazole lauriad
- Mycobutin
- Nascobal
- NebuPen
- nelfinavir
- Neutrexin
- NFV
- Norvir
- Novo-AZT
- Noxafil
- Octagam
- OraQuick
- Oravig
- Panretin
- Paser
- Pentacarinat
- Pentam
- pentamidine
- Peptidic PI
- Pneumopent
- Pneumovax
- Pnu-Imune
- Podofilox
- podophyllin

- posaconazole
- Prezista
- Priftin
- Racivir
- raltegravir
- Rebetron
- Reiki
- Remune
- Rescriptor
- Retrovir
- Reyataz
- Rifadin
- Rifamate
- Rifater
- rilpivirine
- ritonavir
- RO-033-4649
- Roferon A
- saquinavir
- Sculptra
- Selzentry
- Septra
- shikonin
- Sporanox
- stavudine
- Streptomycin sulfate
- Sustiva
- Symmetrel
- Synagis
- T-1249
- tenofovir disoproxil fumarate
- tesamorelin
- tipranavir
- TMC-114
- TMC278
- TNX-355
- Trecator-SC
- trimetrexate

AIDS

- ❑ Trizivir
- ❑ Truvada
- ❑ Valcyte
- ❑ valganciclovir
- ❑ Valtrex
- ❑ Videx
- ❑ Viracept
- ❑ Viramune
- ❑ Viread
- ❑ ViroSe❑ HIV-1
- ❑ Vistide
- ❑ Vitrasert
- ❑ Vitravene
- ❑ Yodoxin
- ❑ zalcitabine
- ❑ Zerit
- ❑ Ziagen
- ❑ zidovudine
- ❑ Zithromax
- ❑ Zithromax Z-Pak
- ❑ Zovirax

ALZHEIMER'S DISEASE

- ❑ ampakine
- ❑ Aricept
- ❑ atomoxetine
- ❑ Cognex
- ❑ Concerta
- ❑ CX-516
- ❑ dexmethylphenidate
- ❑ donepezil
- ❑ Exelon
- ❑ Focalin
- ❑ galantamine Hbr
- ❑ MEM 1414
- ❑ memantine hydrochloride

ALZHEIMER'S DISEASE

- ❑ Metadate
- ❑ Methylin
- ❑ methylphenidate
- ❑ Namenda
- ❑ Phenserine
- ❑ Razadyne
- ❑ Reminyl
- ❑ Riphenidate
- ❑ Ritalin
- ❑ rivastigmine
- ❑ SGS742
- ❑ Strattera
- ❑ Tacrine
- ❑ Trizivir

ANALGESICS

- ❑ abobotulinumtoxinA
- ❑ Abreva
- ❑ Absorbine Jr.
- ❑ Abstral
- ❑ Acephen
- ❑ Aceta
- ❑ acetaminophen
- ❑ Acetavance
- ❑ acrivastine
- ❑ Actamin
- ❑ Actiq
- ❑ Activ On
- ❑ Acubead
- ❑ Acurox
- ❑ Acuvail
- ❑ Adnexsia
- ❑ Advil
- ❑ Advil Liqui-Gels
- ❑ Aflaxin
- ❑ Aggrenox

ANALGESICS

- ❏ Aleve
- ❏ Alfenta
- ❏ alfentanil
- ❏ Alka-Seltzer
- ❏ Allay
- ❏ almotriptan
- ❏ almotriptan malate
- ❏ Alumadrine
- ❏ Amerge
- ❏ Aminofem
- ❏ Anabar
- ❏ Anacin
- ❏ Anakinra
- ❏ Anaprox
- ❏ Anbesol
- ❏ Anexsia
- ❏ aniledrine
- ❏ Anolor
- ❏ Apacet
- ❏ Apamide
- ❏ APAP/Codeine
- ❏ APC
- ❏ Arth Arrest
- ❏ Arth DR
- ❏ Arthrotec
- ❏ Arth-Rx
- ❏ Arthur Itis
- ❏ Ascriptin
- ❏ Aspercreme
- ❏ Aspergum
- ❏ aspirin
- ❏ Astramorph
- ❏ Atasol
- ❏ Atretol
- ❏ Auroto Otic
- ❏ Avinza
- ❏ Axert
- ❏ Axotal

ANALGESICS

- ❏ Azdone
- ❏ Backaid
- ❏ Bactine
- ❏ Bancap
- ❏ Banesin
- ❏ Bayer
- ❏ Benadryl
- ❏ Benadryl-D
- ❏ BeneJoint
- ❏ BENGAY
- ❏ benzocaine
- ❏ Bextra
- ❏ Bicozene
- ❏ Bluboro
- ❏ Bromday
- ❏ bromfenac
- ❏ Bufferin
- ❏ Buffets
- ❏ Bupap
- ❏ Buprenex
- ❏ buprenorphine
- ❏ butalbital
- ❏ butorphanol
- ❏ Butrans
- ❏ Caldolor
- ❏ Cambia
- ❏ Campho-Phenique
- ❏ capsaicin
- ❏ Capzasin-HP
- ❏ carbamazepine
- ❏ Carbatrol
- ❏ carispoprodol
- ❏ Carmex
- ❏ Castiva Arthritis
- ❏ Cataflam
- ❏ Celebrex
- ❏ Cellegisic
- ❏ Cepacol

ANALGESICS

- Cetacaine
- Chloraseptic
- chlorzoxazone
- Clinoril
- clonidine
- Cobroxin
- Codamine
- codeine
- Codrex
- Co-Gesic
- Combunox
- Compoz
- Comtrex
- Congespirin
- Coricidin
- Cox-2 inhibitor
- Dalgan
- Damason
- Dapa
- Darvocet-A 500
- Darvocet-N
- Darvon
- Datril
- Daypro
- Demerol
- DepoDur
- DepoFoam
- Depomorphine
- dezocine
- diclofenac
- diflunisal
- difluprednate
- Dilaudid
- Disalcid
- Doan's
- Dolobid
- Dolacet
- Dolagesic

ANALGESICS

- Dolene-AP
- Dolorac
- Dristan
- Drocade/Aspirin
- Doublecap
- Duraclon
- Duract
- Duragesic
- Duramorph
- Durezol
- Dyloject
- Dysport
- Easprin
- EC-Naprosyn
- Ecotrin
- E-Lor
- Embeda
- Emcodeine
- Empirin
- Empracet
- Emtec
- Enbrel
- Endocet
- enteric aspirin
- Equagesic
- ESGIC
- etanercept
- ethyl aminobenzoate
- etodolac
- etodolic acid
- Exalgo
- Exalgo ER
- Excedrin
- Excedrin Quicktabs
- Exdol
- Exparel
- Extendryl
- EZ III

ANALGESICS

- ☐ Ezol
- ☐ Feldene
- ☐ felodipine
- ☐ Femcet
- ☐ fentanyl
- ☐ fentanyl citrate
- ☐ Fentora
- ☐ Feridex I.V.
- ☐ ferrous fumarate
- ☐ ferrous gluconate
- ☐ ferrous sulfate
- ☐ ferumoxides
- ☐ Feverall
- ☐ fexofenadine
- ☐ Fiberall
- ☐ Fiber-Lax
- ☐ filgrastim
- ☐ Finasteride
- ☐ Fioricet
- ☐ Fiorinal
- ☐ Fiortal
- ☐ Flagyl
- ☐ Flatulex
- ☐ flavoxate
- ☐ flecainide
- ☐ Flector
- ☐ Fleet Babylax
- ☐ Fleet Bisacodyl
- ☐ Fleet Enema
- ☐ Fleet Phospho Soda
- ☐ Flexall
- ☐ Flexaphen
- ☐ Flo-Coat
- ☐ floctafenine
- ☐ Flolan
- ☐ Flomax
- ☐ Flonase
- ☐ Florone

ANALGESICS

- ☐ Flovent
- ☐ Floxan
- ☐ floxuridine
- ☐ Flubiprofen
- ☐ fluconazole
- ☐ flucytosine
- ☐ fludarabine
- ☐ fludrocortisone
- ☐ flumazenil
- ☐ flunisolide
- ☐ fluocinolone
- ☐ fluocinonide
- ☐ Fluogen
- ☐ Fluonid
- ☐ Fluoracaine
- ☐ fluorescein
- ☐ fluoride
- ☐ fluorometholone
- ☐ fluorouracil
- ☐ Fluothane
- ☐ fluoxetine
- ☐ fluoxymesterone
- ☐ fluphenazine
- ☐ flurazepam
- ☐ flurbiprofen
- ☐ Fluress
- ☐ flutamide
- ☐ fluticasone
- ☐ fluvastatin
- ☐ fluvoxamine
- ☐ Fluzone
- ☐ Frova
- ☐ frovatriptan
- ☐ FUDR
- ☐ gaba analog
- ☐ Gelprin
- ☐ Genapap
- ☐ glycyrrhetinic acid

ANALGESICS

- ❏ Goody's
- ❏ Halfprin
- ❏ Head On
- ❏ Healthprin
- ❏ Heet liniment
- ❏ Herpecin-L
- ❏ Hyalgan
- ❏ Hycet
- ❏ Hycomed
- ❏ Hycomine
- ❏ Hycopap
- ❏ Hydrocet
- ❏ hydrocodone bitartrate
- ❏ hydrocodone polistirex
- ❏ Hydrogesic
- ❏ hydromorphone
- ❏ HY-PHEN
- ❏ ibuprofen
- ❏ Icy Hot
- ❏ Indocin
- ❏ Infumorph
- ❏ Ionsys transdermal
- ❏ Ironman
- ❏ JointFlex
- ❏ Kadian
- ❏ Kank-A
- ❏ ketoprolac
- ❏ ketorolac tromethamine
- ❏ Kineret
- ❏ Kneerelief
- ❏ Kolephrin
- ❏ L.M.X.4 cream
- ❏ L.M.X.5 cream
- ❏ Lanotec/Codeine
- ❏ Laudanum
- ❏ Legatrin
- ❏ Leritine
- ❏ Levo-Dromoran

ANALGESICS

- ❏ levophanol
- ❏ Levoprome
- ❏ Lexidronam
- ❏ lidocaine
- ❏ Lidoderm patch
- ❏ Liquiprin
- ❏ Lodine
- ❏ Lorcet
- ❏ Lortab
- ❏ Lurline
- ❏ Lyrica
- ❏ Margesic
- ❏ Maxalt-MLT
- ❏ Max-Freeze
- ❏ Maxidone
- ❏ Medastron
- ❏ Medigesic
- ❏ mefenamic acid
- ❏ Mepergan
- ❏ Meperidine
- ❏ meprobamate
- ❏ Methadone
- ❏ Midol
- ❏ Midrin
- ❏ MigraHealth
- ❏ Migra spray
- ❏ milnacipran
- ❏ Mobigesic
- ❏ Mono-Gesic
- ❏ morphine sulfate
- ❏ Motrin
- ❏ MoxDuo IR
- ❏ MS Contin
- ❏ MSIR
- ❏ MT100
- ❏ Myoflex
- ❏ nalbuphine
- ❏ Nalfon

ANALGESICS

- ❏ naloxone
- ❏ naltrexone hydrochloride
- ❏ Naprelan
- ❏ Naprosyn
- ❏ naratriptan
- ❏ NasalFent
- ❏ Neopap
- ❏ nepafenac
- ❏ Neurontin
- ❏ Nevanac
- ❏ Norco
- ❏ Norel
- ❏ Norflex
- ❏ Norgesic
- ❏ Novitra
- ❏ Novo-AC
- ❏ Novogesic
- ❏ Nubain
- ❏ Nucofed
- ❏ Nucynta
- ❏ Numorphan
- ❏ Nupercainal
- ❏ Ofirmev
- ❏ Onset
- ❏ Onsolis
- ❏ Opana
- ❏ Orabase
- ❏ Orajel
- ❏ Oramorph
- ❏ Oraphen
- ❏ OraVescent Fentanyl
- ❏ Orlamm
- ❏ Ornex
- ❏ orphenadrine
- ❏ orphengesic
- ❏ Orudis
- ❏ Oruvail
- ❏ Oxecta

ANALGESICS

- ❏ Oxycet
- ❏ Oxycodan
- ❏ oxycodone
- ❏ OxyContin
- ❏ Oxy-Fast
- ❏ Oxy-IR
- ❏ oxymorphone
- ❏ Pacaps
- ❏ PainBust-R
- ❏ Palladone
- ❏ Pamprin
- ❏ Panacet
- ❏ Panadol
- ❏ Panasal
- ❏ Panlor
- ❏ Paraflex
- ❏ Parafon Forte
- ❏ PC Cap
- ❏ pentazocine
- ❏ Percocet
- ❏ Percodan
- ❏ Percogesic
- ❏ Percolone
- ❏ Perform
- ❏ Phenaphen/Codeine
- ❏ Phenergan
- ❏ phenol
- ❏ Phrenilin Forte
- ❏ Polygesic
- ❏ Ponstel
- ❏ Pregabalin
- ❏ Premsyn
- ❏ Prialt
- ❏ Prid
- ❏ Prodium
- ❏ Propacet
- ❏ Pro Pox/APAP
- ❏ propoxyphene

ANALGESICS

- ❑ propoxyphene napsylate
- ❑ Protid
- ❑ Pyregesic
- ❑ Pyridium
- ❑ Quadramet
- ❑ Qutenza
- ❑ Ralivia
- ❑ Rapinyl
- ❑ Rectiv
- ❑ Redutemp
- ❑ Relafen
- ❑ Releev
- ❑ Remoxy
- ❑ Repan
- ❑ Relpax
- ❑ Rid-A-Pain
- ❑ Robaxin
- ❑ rofecoxib
- ❑ ROX-888
- ❑ Roxanol
- ❑ Roxicet
- ❑ Roxicodone
- ❑ Roxiflex
- ❑ Roxilox
- ❑ Roxiprin
- ❑ Ryzolt
- ❑ St. Joseph Aspirin
- ❑ Saleto
- ❑ Salflex
- ❑ Salonpas
- ❑ Sansert
- ❑ Sativex
- ❑ Sedapap
- ❑ Semprex
- ❑ Sinarest
- ❑ Sine-Aid
- ❑ Sinulin
- ❑ Sinutab

ANALGESICS

- ❑ Snaplets
- ❑ Soma Compound
- ❑ Sprix
- ❑ Stadol
- ❑ Stagesic
- ❑ Stanback
- ❑ Stopain
- ❑ Sublimaze
- ❑ Sudafed
- ❑ Sufenta
- ❑ sufentanil
- ❑ sumatriptan
- ❑ Sumavel DosePro
- ❑ Sunril
- ❑ Supac
- ❑ Suppap
- ❑ Synalgos
- ❑ Synvisc
- ❑ Talacen
- ❑ Talwin
- ❑ Tanac
- ❑ Tapanol
- ❑ tapentadol
- ❑ Tegretol
- ❑ Tempra
- ❑ Tencon
- ❑ Theragesic
- ❑ ThermaCare
- ❑ Tiger Balm
- ❑ Tolectin
- ❑ Topricin
- ❑ Toradol
- ❑ Tramadol
- ❑ Tranadik
- ❑ Traumeel
- ❑ Trexima
- ❑ Treximet
- ❑ Trilisate

ANALGESICS

- ❑ Tylaprin/Codeine
- ❑ Tylenol
- ❑ Tylenol caplets
- ❑ Tylenol geltabs
- ❑ Tylox
- ❑ Ugesic
- ❑ Ultiva
- ❑ Ultracet
- ❑ Ultragesic
- ❑ Ulram
- ❑ Uniserts
- ❑ Ursinus
- ❑ valdecoxib
- ❑ Valorin
- ❑ Vanacet
- ❑ Vanquish
- ❑ Vapocet
- ❑ Veganin
- ❑ Vendone
- ❑ Vicodin
- ❑ Vicoprofen
- ❑ Vioxx
- ❑ ViTelle Lurline PMS
- ❑ Voltaren
- ❑ Wygesic
- ❑ XiDay
- ❑ Zebutal
- ❑ Zeel
- ❑ Zelrix
- ❑ Zilactin
- ❑ Zingo
- ❑ Zipsor
- ❑ Zostrix
- ❑ Zydone

ANESTHETICS

- ❑ Abstral
- ❑ Akten

ANESTHETICS

- ❑ Americaine
- ❑ Amidate
- ❑ Amytal
- ❑ Anectine
- ❑ Anestacon
- ❑ aniledrine
- ❑ Aquachloral
- ❑ Aquavan
- ❑ Aramine
- ❑ Articaine
- ❑ Astracaine
- ❑ atracurium
- ❑ Avertin
- ❑ Bactine
- ❑ benzocaine
- ❑ Benzodent
- ❑ Blockain
- ❑ brevital, sodium
- ❑ Brietal
- ❑ bupivacaine
- ❑ Butadiene
- ❑ Carbocaine
- ❑ Cetacaine
- ❑ Chirocaine
- ❑ chloral hydrate
- ❑ chloroethane
- ❑ chloroform
- ❑ chloroprocaine
- ❑ cisatracurium besylate
- ❑ Citanest
- ❑ curare
- ❑ Cyclaine
- ❑ cyclohexane
- ❑ cyclopentane
- ❑ cyclopropane
- ❑ Dalcaine
- ❑ Dentapaine
- ❑ Dent-Zel-Ite
- ❑ desflurane

ANESTHETICS

- diethyl ether
- Diprivan
- divinyl oxide
- doxacurium
- doxapram
- Droperidol
- Duranest
- Dyclone
- dyclonine
- EMLA
- enflurane
- ether
- Ethocaine
- Ethrane
- ethyl aminobenzoate
- Ethylene
- ethyl ether
- etidocaine
- fentanyl
- Fleet Anorectal
- flumazenil
- flunitrazepam
- Fluothane
- Fluro-Ethyl
- Forane
- fospropofol
- Halothane
- Hemorid
- Hexylcaine
- Hurricaine
- Innovar
- Inapsine
- Iontophoretic
- Isocaine
- isoflurane
- Ketalar
- L-Caine
- Lanacane
- Leritine

ANESTHETICS

- levobupivacaine
- lidocaine
- Lidoject
- LidoSite
- Lusedra
- Marcaine
- Mepergan
- meperidine
- mepivacaine
- metaraminol
- methohexital
- methoxamine
- midazolam
- Mivacron
- mivacurium
- Naropin
- Nesacaine
- Nimbex
- Noctec
- Norcuron
- Novocain
- novochlorhydrate
- Numzident
- Num-Zit-Gel
- Nupercainal
- Nuromax
- Octocaine
- On-Q
- Ophthaine
- Oraqix
- OraVerse
- pancuronium
- Pavulon
- Penthrane
- Polocaine
- Pontocaine
- Preject
- Preparation H
- prilocaine

ANESTHETICS

- [ ] procaine
- [ ] ProctoFoam
- [ ] propofo
- [ ] Rapinyl
- [ ] Raplon
- [ ] remifentanil
- [ ] Robinul
- [ ] rocuronium
- [ ] Rohypnol
- [ ] Romazicon
- [ ] ropivacaine
- [ ] Sarapin
- [ ] S-Caine Peel
- [ ] Sensorcaine
- [ ] Sevoflurane
- [ ] sodium brevital
- [ ] sodium pentothal
- [ ] Sojourn Sevoflurane
- [ ] Solarcaine
- [ ] Sublimaze
- [ ] succinylcholine
- [ ] Suprane
- [ ] surital sodium
- [ ] Synera
- [ ] tetracaine
- [ ] thiopental sodium
- [ ] Tracrium
- [ ] Tronolane
- [ ] Tucks
- [ ] Ultane
- [ ] Ultiva
- [ ] Ultracaine
- [ ] Vasoxyl
- [ ] vecuronium
- [ ] Versed
- [ ] Xylocaine
- [ ] Zemuron
- [ ] Zilactin

ANTACIDS

- [ ] AcipHex
- [ ] Alka-Seltzer
- [ ] Alternagel
- [ ] aluminum hydroxide
- [ ] aluminum magnesia
- [ ] Amitone
- [ ] Amphojel
- [ ] Axid
- [ ] Beano
- [ ] Beano Meltaways
- [ ] bethanechol
- [ ] Bisodol
- [ ] Brioschi Powder
- [ ] calcium carbonate
- [ ] Camalox
- [ ] Carafate
- [ ] Carbamine
- [ ] Ceo Two
- [ ] CharcoCaps
- [ ] Chooz
- [ ] cimetidine
- [ ] citrocarbonate
- [ ] Dexilant
- [ ] dexlansoprazole
- [ ] Dicarbosil
- [ ] Di-Gel
- [ ] Duexa
- [ ] esomeprazole magnesium
- [ ] Famodine
- [ ] famotidine
- [ ] Fluxid
- [ ] GasAid
- [ ] Gas-X
- [ ] Gaviscon
- [ ] Gelcid
- [ ] Gelusil
- [ ] H2 Blockers
- [ ] Kapidex

ANTACIDS

- ❑ Kolantyl
- ❑ Kudrox
- ❑ lansoprazole
- ❑ Little Tummys
- ❑ Maalox
- ❑ Mag-al
- ❑ Magnatril
- ❑ magnesium carbonate
- ❑ magnesium hydroxide
- ❑ magnesium oxide
- ❑ magnesium trisilicate
- ❑ metoclopramide
- ❑ Metozolv ODT
- ❑ Milk of Magnesia
- ❑ Mylanta
- ❑ Mylicon
- ❑ Nephrox
- ❑ Neutrolox
- ❑ Nexium
- ❑ Nulev
- ❑ omeprazole
- ❑ Oxaine
- ❑ pantoprazole
- ❑ pentagastrin
- ❑ Pepcid
- ❑ Pepcid AC
- ❑ Peptavlon
- ❑ Pepto-Bismol
- ❑ Pepto-Bismol Max
- ❑ Pepto-Bismol InstaCool
- ❑ Phazyme
- ❑ Phillips Milk of Magnesia
- ❑ PN 400
- ❑ Prevacid
- ❑ Prilosec
- ❑ Prilosec OTC
- ❑ prokinetics
- ❑ Protonix

ANTACIDS

- ❑ proton pump inhibitors
- ❑ rabeprazole
- ❑ ranitidine
- ❑ Rapinex
- ❑ Reglan
- ❑ Riopan
- ❑ Rolaids
- ❑ Rolaids softchews
- ❑ sucralftate
- ❑ Tagamet
- ❑ Tegaserod
- ❑ Titralac
- ❑ Tums
- ❑ Urecholine
- ❑ Vimovo
- ❑ Zantac
- ❑ Zegerid
- ❑ Zegerid OTC
- ❑ Zelnorm

ANTIBIOTICS

- ❑ Achromycin
- ❑ Adoxa
- ❑ Advicor
- ❑ Amikacin
- ❑ Amikin
- ❑ Ancef
- ❑ Ancobon
- ❑ alpha-proteinase
- ❑ anidulafungin
- ❑ Ansamycin
- ❑ Antibiopto
- ❑ Aralast NP
- ❑ Arcalyst
- ❑ atovaquone
- ❑ Atrosept

ANTIBIOTICS

- ❑ Augmentin
- ❑ Aureomycin
- ❑ Avelox
- ❑ Azactam
- ❑ azafluoroquinolone
- ❑ AzaSite
- ❑ azithromycin
- ❑ aztreonam
- ❑ aztreonam lysine
- ❑ bacampicillin
- ❑ Bacitracin
- ❑ Bactine
- ❑ Bactocill
- ❑ Bactrim
- ❑ besifloxacin
- ❑ Besivance
- ❑ beta-lactame
- ❑ Biaxin
- ❑ Bicillin
- ❑ Biocef
- ❑ Bio-Triple
- ❑ biskalcitrate
- ❑ Blenoxane
- ❑ bleomycin
- ❑ Bleph-10
- ❑ Cancidas
- ❑ Capastat
- ❑ capreomycin
- ❑ carbenicillin indanyl
- ❑ caspofungin
- ❑ Cayston
- ❑ Ceclor
- ❑ Cedax
- ❑ cefaclor
- ❑ Cefadyl
- ❑ cefadroxil
- ❑ cefamandole naftate
- ❑ cefazolin

ANTIBIOTICS

- ❑ cefdinir
- ❑ cefditoren
- ❑ cefepime
- ❑ cefixime
- ❑ Cefotan
- ❑ cefotaxime
- ❑ cefotetan disodium
- ❑ cefoxitin
- ❑ cefpodoxime
- ❑ cefprozil
- ❑ ceftaroline fosamil
- ❑ ceftazidime
- ❑ ceftibuten
- ❑ Ceftin
- ❑ ceftizoxime
- ❑ Ceftobiprole
- ❑ ceftriaxone
- ❑ cefuroxime
- ❑ cefzil
- ❑ cephalexin
- ❑ cephalosporin
- ❑ Cephalothin
- ❑ Cephapirin
- ❑ cephradine
- ❑ Ceptaz
- ❑ Cerubidine
- ❑ cethromycin
- ❑ Cetraxal
- ❑ Chibroxin
- ❑ chloramphenicol
- ❑ Chloromycetin
- ❑ Chlorocol
- ❑ Chlorofair
- ❑ Chloroptic
- ❑ Cidomycin
- ❑ Ciloxan
- ❑ Cinobac
- ❑ cinoxacin

ANTIBIOTICS

- ❑ Cipro
- ❑ ciprofloxacin
- ❑ Claforan
- ❑ clarithromycin
- ❑ Cleocin
- ❑ Clindagel
- ❑ Cloxacillin
- ❑ Cloxapen
- ❑ colistimethate
- ❑ Colistin
- ❑ Coly-Mycin
- ❑ Cosmegen
- ❑ dactinomycin
- ❑ Daflopristin
- ❑ Daraprim
- ❑ DaunoXome
- ❑ Declomycin
- ❑ demeclocycline
- ❑ dicloxacillin
- ❑ Dificid
- ❑ Diflucan
- ❑ dirithromycin
- ❑ DisperMox
- ❑ Dolsed
- ❑ Doribax
- ❑ doripenem
- ❑ Doryx
- ❑ Doxil
- ❑ doxorubicin
- ❑ doxycycline calcium
- ❑ doxycycline hyclate
- ❑ doxycycline monohydrate
- ❑ Dual
- ❑ Duricef
- ❑ Dycill
- ❑ Dynabac
- ❑ Dynacin
- ❑ Dynapen

ANTIBIOTICS

- ❑ Econochlor
- ❑ E-Mycin
- ❑ enoxacin
- ❑ E.E.S.
- ❑ ertapenem
- ❑ Eryc
- ❑ Ery-Ped
- ❑ Ery-Tab
- ❑ Erythrocin
- ❑ erythromycin ethylsuccinate
- ❑ Eryzole
- ❑ Factive
- ❑ Femguard
- ❑ Fenicol
- ❑ fidaxomicin
- ❑ Flagyl
- ❑ Floxin
- ❑ fluconazole
- ❑ flucytosine
- ❑ fluoroquinolone
- ❑ fomivirsen
- ❑ Fortaz
- ❑ fosfomycin
- ❑ Fulvicin
- ❑ Furadantin
- ❑ Furalan
- ❑ Furan
- ❑ Furanite
- ❑ furazolidone
- ❑ Furoxone
- ❑ fusidic acid
- ❑ Gantrisin
- ❑ Garamycin
- ❑ gatifloxacin
- ❑ gemifloxacin mesylate
- ❑ Genoptic
- ❑ Gentacidin
- ❑ Gentafair

ANTIBIOTICS

- Gentak
- gentamycin
- Gentrasul
- Geocillin
- Geopen
- G-Myticin
- Gramicidin
- grepafloxacin
- Grisactin
- griseofulvin
- Gris-PEG
- Gyne-Sulf
- Helizide
- Herpetrol
- Hiprex
- Iclaprim
- Idamycin
- Ilosone
- Ilotycin
- imipenem
- Invanz
- Iquix
- Jenamicin
- Kanamycin
- Kantrex
- Keflex
- Keftab
- Kefurox
- Kefzol
- Kenalog
- Ketek
- ketoconazole
- Lamisil
- lansoprazole
- Levaquin
- Levofloxacin
- Lincocin
- linezolid
- linosamides

ANTIBIOTICS

- lomefloxacin
- Lorabid
- loracarbef
- Loridine
- Lyphocin
- Macrobid
- Macrodantin
- macrolide
- mandelamine
- Mandol
- Maximime
- Maxaquin
- Mefoxin
- Menactra
- Mepron
- meropenem
- Merrem
- methenamine
- metronidazole
- Mezlin
- mezlocillin
- micafungin
- Minocin
- minocycline
- Mithracin
- Mitomycin
- Monocid
- Monodox
- Monurol
- Moxatag
- Moxeza
- moxifloxacin
- Mutamycin
- Mycamine
- Mycobutin
- Mycolog
- Nafcillin
- nalidixic acid
- Nebcin

ANTIBIOTICS

- ☐ NegGram
- ☐ Neocidin
- ☐ NeoDecadron
- ☐ neomycin
- ☐ Neosporin
- ☐ Neotal
- ☐ Neotricin
- ☐ Netromycin
- ☐ Neutrexin
- ☐ Nipent
- ☐ nitrofurantoin
- ☐ norfloxacin
- ☐ Noroxin
- ☐ Novantrone
- ☐ Noxafil
- ☐ Nystatin
- ☐ Ocu-Chlor
- ☐ Ocuflox
- ☐ Ocu-Mycin
- ☐ Ocu-Spor
- ☐ Ocu-Sulf
- ☐ Ocutricin
- ☐ ofloxacin
- ☐ oleandomycin
- ☐ Omnicef
- ☐ Omnipen
- ☐ Ophthacet
- ☐ oxacillin
- ☐ oxytetracycline
- ☐ Pathocil
- ☐ PCE
- ☐ Pediazole
- ☐ Penetrex
- ☐ penicillin
- ☐ Pentamycetin
- ☐ Pen-Vee
- ☐ peptides
- ☐ peptolides
- ☐ Permapen

ANTIBIOTICS

- ☐ Pfizerpen
- ☐ phosphomycin
- ☐ piperacillin
- ☐ Pipracil
- ☐ Plexion
- ☐ P.N. Ophthalmic
- ☐ polymyxin
- ☐ polypeptide
- ☐ Polysporin
- ☐ Polytrim
- ☐ posaconazole
- ☐ Prevpac
- ☐ Primaxin
- ☐ Primsol
- ☐ Proloprim
- ☐ Pylera
- ☐ quinolone
- ☐ Raxar
- ☐ Regasporin
- ☐ Restanza
- ☐ rifabutin
- ☐ Rifadin
- ☐ Rifamate
- ☐ rifampin
- ☐ Rifatar
- ☐ rifaximin
- ☐ rilonacept
- ☐ Rocephin
- ☐ Rovamycine
- ☐ Rubex
- ☐ Septra
- ☐ Seromycin
- ☐ sodium sulamyd
- ☐ Sopramycetin
- ☐ sparfloxacin
- ☐ spectinomycin
- ☐ Spectracef
- ☐ Spectrobid
- ☐ Spectro-Chlor

ANTIBIOTICS

- ❑ Spectro-Genta
- ❑ Spectro-Sporin
- ❑ Spectro-Sulf
- ❑ spiramycin
- ❑ Sporanox
- ❑ Staticin
- ❑ Streptomycin
- ❑ Sulf 10
- ❑ sulfacetamide
- ❑ sulfacytine
- ❑ sulfadiazine
- ❑ sulfabenzamide
- ❑ Sulfa-Gyn
- ❑ Sulfair
- ❑ sulfamethoprim
- ❑ sulfamethoxazole
- ❑ Sulfamide
- ❑ Sulfatrim
- ❑ Sulfa-Trip
- ❑ Sulfex
- ❑ sulfisoxazole
- ❑ sulfonamide
- ❑ Sumycin
- ❑ Suprax
- ❑ Synercid
- ❑ TAO
- ❑ Tazicef
- ❑ Tazidime
- ❑ Teflaro
- ❑ telavancin
- ❑ telithromycin
- ❑ Tequin
- ❑ Terra-Cortril
- ❑ Terramycin
- ❑ tetracycline
- ❑ Ticar
- ❑ ticarcillin
- ❑ Tifacogin
- ❑ tigecycline

ANTIBIOTICS

- ❑ Timentin
- ❑ Tindamax
- ❑ tinidazole
- ❑ TOBI
- ❑ TobraDex
- ❑ Tobramycin
- ❑ triamcinolone
- ❑ Tribiotic
- ❑ trimethoprim
- ❑ Trimpex
- ❑ Tri-Ophthalmic
- ❑ Tri-Thalmic
- ❑ troleandomycin
- ❑ Trovan
- ❑ Trysul
- ❑ T-Stat
- ❑ Tygacil
- ❑ Unasyn
- ❑ Urex
- ❑ Uricalm
- ❑ Urised
- ❑ Urobiotic
- ❑ Uroplus
- ❑ Uroquid
- ❑ Valstar
- ❑ Vancocin
- ❑ Vancoled
- ❑ vancomycin
- ❑ Vantin
- ❑ Vectrin
- ❑ Veetids
- ❑ Velosef
- ❑ Vibativ
- ❑ Vibramycin
- ❑ Vigtravene
- ❑ Viroptic
- ❑ Wycillin
- ❑ Wymox
- ❑ Xifaxan

ANTIBIOTICS

- ❏ Xigris
- ❏ Zartan
- ❏ Zefazone
- ❏ Zinacef
- ❏ Zithromax
- ❏ Zithromax Z-Pak
- ❏ Zmax
- ❏ Zolicef
- ❏ Zosyn
- ❏ Zotrim
- ❏ Zygam
- ❏ Zymaxid
- ❏ Zyvox

ANTI-COAGULANTS

- ❏ Abbokinase
- ❏ Abbokinase Open-Cath
- ❏ Acenocoumarol
- ❏ acetylsalicylic acid
- ❏ alteplase
- ❏ Ancrod
- ❏ Angiomax
- ❏ Anisindione
- ❏ argatroban
- ❏ Arixtra
- ❏ Ascriptin
- ❏ aspirin
- ❏ bivalirudin
- ❏ Bufferin
- ❏ calciparine
- ❏ Cathflo Activase
- ❏ Coumadin
- ❏ dalteparin
- ❏ danaparoid
- ❏ Dicumarol
- ❏ dipyridamole

ANTI-COAGULANTS

- ❏ enoxaparin
- ❏ enteric aspirin
- ❏ Exanta
- ❏ fondaparinux
- ❏ Fragmin
- ❏ Heparin
- ❏ Kabikinase
- ❏ Lepirudin
- ❏ Liquaemin
- ❏ Lovenox
- ❏ Miradon
- ❏ Normiflo
- ❏ Orgaran
- ❏ Persantine
- ❏ Refludan
- ❏ Sintrom
- ❏ TPA
- ❏ Urokinase
- ❏ warfarin
- ❏ ximelagatran

ANTIDOTES

- ❏ acamprosate
- ❏ Acetadote
- ❏ acetylcysteine
- ❏ Actidose
- ❏ Actidose-Aqua
- ❏ activated charcoal
- ❏ amyl nitrate
- ❏ Anascorp
- ❏ Antabuse
- ❏ Antilirium
- ❏ Antizol
- ❏ ATNNA
- ❏ Atropen
- ❏ BAL in oil

ANTIDOTES

- calcium disodium
- Campral
- catapres
- Centruroides
- Chantix
- chelating agents
- Chemet
- citrovorum factor
- Cuprimine
- Cyanokit
- deferiprone
- deferoxamine mesylate
- Desferal
- Depade
- Depen
- Digibind
- Digoxin
- dimercaprol
- disulfiram
- Edecrin
- ethacrynic acid
- Ferriprox
- flumazenil
- folinic acid
- fomepizole
- Fusilev
- Habitrol
- hydroxocobalamin
- Isovorin
- leucovorin rescue
- levoleucovorin
- Liqui-Char
- magnesium sulfate
- methylene blue
- Mucomyst
- Mucosil
- nalmefene
- naloxone
- naltrexone

ANTIDOTES

- Narcan
- NicoDerm CQ
- Nicorette
- Penicillamine
- physostigmine
- pralidoxime chloride
- protamine sulfate
- Protopam chloride
- pyridoxine
- Revex
- ReVia
- Romazicon
- sodium nitrate
- sodium thiosulfate
- Suboxone
- Subutex
- succimer
- Trexan
- universal
- Urolene Blue
- varenicline
- Vivitrex
- Vivitrol
- Wellcovorin

ANTI-EMETICS

- Aloxi
- Antivert
- Anzemet
- APF530
- Arrestin
- Atarax
- Benadryl
- Benadryl-D
- Bendectin
- Benzacot
- Bonine

ANTI-EMETICS

- ❏ Bucladin-S
- ❏ Cesamet
- ❏ Chaser Plus
- ❏ chlorpromazine
- ❏ Compazine
- ❏ Cyclizine
- ❏ diphenhydramine
- ❏ dolasetron
- ❏ Dramamine
- ❏ dronabinol
- ❏ droperidol
- ❏ Elavil
- ❏ Emecheck
- ❏ Emend
- ❏ Emesert
- ❏ Emetrol
- ❏ fosaprepitant dimeglumine
- ❏ granisetron
- ❏ Hyoscine
- ❏ Kytril
- ❏ Little Tummys
- ❏ lorazepam
- ❏ Marezine
- ❏ Marinol
- ❏ Maxeran
- ❏ meclizine
- ❏ Mepergan
- ❏ metoclopramide
- ❏ midocrine
- ❏ MT100
- ❏ Nabilone
- ❏ Nausetrol
- ❏ Nauzene
- ❏ Netupitant
- ❏ Octamide PFS
- ❏ ondansetron
- ❏ palonosetron
- ❏ perphenazine
- ❏ Phenergan

ANTI-EMETICS

- ❏ ProAmatine
- ❏ prochlorperazine
- ❏ promethazine
- ❏ pyridoxine
- ❏ Reglan
- ❏ Sancuso
- ❏ scopolamine
- ❏ Sea-Band
- ❏ Stemetic
- ❏ Tebamide
- ❏ thiethylperazine
- ❏ Thorazine
- ❏ Ticon
- ❏ Tigan
- ❏ Torecan
- ❏ Transderm SCOP
- ❏ Triban
- ❏ Tribenzagan
- ❏ Trilafon
- ❏ trimethobenzamide
- ❏ Vertigoheel
- ❏ Vistaril
- ❏ Zentrip
- ❏ Zofran
- ❏ Zontrol
- ❏ Zuplenz

ANTI-INFLAMMATORY

- ❏ acetaminophen
- ❏ Acetavance
- ❏ Acular
- ❏ Acuvail
- ❏ Advil
- ❏ Aerobid
- ❏ AK-Pred
- ❏ AK-Tate
- ❏ Alka-Butazolidin

ANTI-INFLAMMATORY

- ❑ Alkabutazone
- ❑ Alrex
- ❑ Amersol
- ❑ Anaprox
- ❑ Ansaid
- ❑ Apsifen
- ❑ Arcalyst
- ❑ Arthrotec
- ❑ Asacol
- ❑ Azmacort
- ❑ Azulfidine
- ❑ Baldex
- ❑ balsalazide
- ❑ Beclovent
- ❑ betamethasone
- ❑ betamethasone dipropionate
- ❑ betamethasone valerate
- ❑ Betnesol
- ❑ Bromday
- ❑ bromfenac
- ❑ Bufferin
- ❑ butazolidin
- ❑ C1 Inhibitor
- ❑ Caldolor
- ❑ Cambia
- ❑ Cataflam
- ❑ Celebrex
- ❑ certolizumab pegol
- ❑ Cimzia
- ❑ Cinryze
- ❑ Clinoril
- ❑ Colazal
- ❑ Cordran
- ❑ Cortemed
- ❑ cortisol
- ❑ cortisone
- ❑ Cortisporin
- ❑ Cutivate

ANTI-INFLAMMATORY

- ❑ D2E7
- ❑ Dalalone
- ❑ Daypro
- ❑ Decacort
- ❑ Decadron
- ❑ Depo-Medrol
- ❑ DesOwen
- ❑ dexair
- ❑ dexamethasone
- ❑ Dexotic
- ❑ Dexsone
- ❑ diclofenac
- ❑ diclofenac potassium
- ❑ diflunisal
- ❑ difluprednate
- ❑ Diodex
- ❑ Dipentum
- ❑ Diprolene
- ❑ Disalcid
- ❑ Doan's pills
- ❑ Dolobid
- ❑ Duract
- ❑ Durezol
- ❑ Dyloject
- ❑ EC-Naprosyn
- ❑ Econopred
- ❑ Eflone
- ❑ enteric aspirin
- ❑ Feldene
- ❑ fenoprofen
- ❑ Flarex
- ❑ flavocoxid
- ❑ floctafenine
- ❑ Flo-Pred
- ❑ Flovent
- ❑ fluorometholone
- ❑ flurbiprofen
- ❑ Flur-Op

ANTI-INFLAMMATORY

- ❏ Haltran
- ❏ hydrocortisone
- ❏ Ibren
- ❏ IBU
- ❏ Ibuprin
- ❏ ibuprofen
- ❏ ibuprofen lysine
- ❏ Ibuprohm
- ❏ Ibu-Tab
- ❏ Indocin
- ❏ indomethacin
- ❏ Inflamase
- ❏ I-Pred
- ❏ ketoprofen
- ❏ ketorolac tromethamine
- ❏ Lidex
- ❏ Life-Pred
- ❏ Limbrel
- ❏ Lipsovir
- ❏ Lodine
- ❏ Lotemax
- ❏ loteprednol
- ❏ LSAIDS
- ❏ Luxig
- ❏ Lysine
- ❏ Magan
- ❏ magnesium salicylate
- ❏ Magsal
- ❏ Maxidex
- ❏ Meclomen
- ❏ Medipren
- ❏ medrysone
- ❏ mefenamic acid
- ❏ meflofenamate
- ❏ meloxicam
- ❏ mesalamine
- ❏ methylprednisolone
- ❏ Midol

ANTI-INFLAMMATORY

- ❏ Mobic
- ❏ Mobidin
- ❏ Motrin
- ❏ nabumetone
- ❏ Nalfon
- ❏ Naprelan
- ❏ Naprosyn
- ❏ naproxcinod
- ❏ Naproxen
- ❏ NeoDecadron
- ❏ NeoProfen
- ❏ nepafenac
- ❏ Nevanac
- ❏ NSAIDS
- ❏ Nuprin
- ❏ Ocu-Dex
- ❏ Ocufen
- ❏ Ocu-Pred
- ❏ olsalaine
- ❏ Orudis
- ❏ Oruvail
- ❏ oxaprozin
- ❏ Pamprin
- ❏ Paxofen
- ❏ Pedia
- ❏ Pennsaid
- ❏ Pentasa
- ❏ phenylbutazone
- ❏ Phenylone Plus
- ❏ piroxicam
- ❏ Ponstan
- ❏ Ponstel
- ❏ Pred Forte
- ❏ prednisolone
- ❏ Prednisone
- ❏ Profenal
- ❏ Progesic
- ❏ pseudopterosin

ANTI-INFLAMMATORY

- ❏ Psorcon
- ❏ Pulmicort
- ❏ Q-Profen
- ❏ Relafen
- ❏ rilonacept
- ❏ rimexolone
- ❏ rofecoxib
- ❏ Rowasa
- ❏ Rufen
- ❏ salsalate
- ❏ Spersadex
- ❏ Storz-Dexa
- ❏ sulfasalazine
- ❏ sulindac
- ❏ sumatriptan
- ❏ Sumavel DosePro
- ❏ Surgam
- ❏ Synflex
- ❏ tenoxicam
- ❏ tiaprofenic acid
- ❏ Tilade
- ❏ Tobradex
- ❏ Tolectin
- ❏ Tolmectin
- ❏ Topricin
- ❏ Toradol
- ❏ Traumeel
- ❏ Trendar
- ❏ Trexima
- ❏ Treximet
- ❏ triamcinolone
- ❏ Trilisate
- ❏ Trivaris
- ❏ Ultra-Pred
- ❏ Ultravate
- ❏ Vancenase
- ❏ Vanceril
- ❏ Vanoxide

ANTI-INFLAMMATORY

- ❏ Vexol
- ❏ Vicuprofen
- ❏ Vimovo
- ❏ Vioxx
- ❏ Voltaren
- ❏ Voltarol
- ❏ Zeel

ANTISEPTICS

- ❏ Abreva
- ❏ Anbesol
- ❏ Bactine
- ❏ benzalkonium
- ❏ Betadine
- ❏ Bithionol
- ❏ Campho-Phenique
- ❏ Castellani
- ❏ Cepacol
- ❏ ChloraPrep
- ❏ Chloraseptic
- ❏ chlorazene
- ❏ chlorhexidine
- ❏ Clorpactin
- ❏ CureChrome
- ❏ Diaparene
- ❏ Guaiacol
- ❏ Halazone
- ❏ Herpecin-L
- ❏ hexachlorophene
- ❏ hexylresorcinol
- ❏ Hibiclens
- ❏ Hibistat
- ❏ hydrogen peroxide
- ❏ iodine
- ❏ isopropyl alcohol
- ❏ Kank-A

ANTISEPTICS

- merbromin
- Mercurochrome
- Merthiolate
- methylparaben
- Novitra
- Orabase
- Orajel
- oxyguinoline salts
- phenol
- pHisoHex
- picric acid
- povidone/iodine
- propylparaban
- Proxacol
- Puri-Clens
- pyrogallol
- Releev
- resorcinol
- Safe 4 Hours
- Tanac
- thimersol
- Thymol
- ULTRACEPT
- Zilactin

ARTHRITIS

- abatacept
- Aclasta
- Actemra
- Acthar Gel
- ACZ885
- adalimumab
- Adlone
- Aflexa
- Aleve
- Alloprim

ARTHRITIS

- allopurinol
- almotriptan
- almotriptan malate
- Amcort
- Anaprox
- Anturane
- Arava
- Aristocort
- Aristospan
- Arthriten
- Arth-Rx
- Ascriptin
- Atolone
- auranofin
- Axert
- Azulfidine
- BeneJoint
- Benemid
- BENGAY
- betamethasone
- Bextra
- BioLon
- Bufferin
- Caldolor
- Castiva Arthritis
- Cataflam
- celecoxib
- Celestone
- Cel-U-Jec injection
- Cerebrex
- chondroitin
- Cimzia
- civamide
- Civanex
- Clinoril
- CM Plex
- ColBENEMID
- colchicine

ARTHRITIS

- ❑ Colcrys
- ❑ corticotropin
- ❑ cortisone
- ❑ Cortone
- ❑ COX-2
- ❑ Cuprimine
- ❑ cyclosporine
- ❑ D2E7
- ❑ DayPro
- ❑ Decadron
- ❑ Decaject
- ❑ Delta-Cortef
- ❑ Deltasone
- ❑ Depen
- ❑ depMedalone
- ❑ Depoject
- ❑ Depo-Medrol
- ❑ dexamethasone
- ❑ Dexasone
- ❑ Dexone
- ❑ diclofenac
- ❑ Diflunisal
- ❑ Diopred
- ❑ Disalcid
- ❑ D-Med injection
- ❑ Dolobid
- ❑ Duexis
- ❑ Duralone
- ❑ Easprin
- ❑ EC-Naprosyn
- ❑ efalizumab
- ❑ Elaprase
- ❑ Enbrel
- ❑ esomeprazole magnesium
- ❑ etanercept
- ❑ etodolac
- ❑ Feldene
- ❑ fenoprofen

ARTHRITIS

- ❑ flavocoxid
- ❑ Flexable
- ❑ Flexamin
- ❑ Flexanew
- ❑ Flexium
- ❑ Folex PFS
- ❑ glucosamine
- ❑ golimumab
- ❑ Haldrone
- ❑ Hexadrol
- ❑ H.P. Acthar Gel
- ❑ Humira
- ❑ Hyalgan
- ❑ Hyaluronate
- ❑ Hydeltra
- ❑ Hydeltrasol
- ❑ hydrocortisone
- ❑ IBU
- ❑ ibuprofen
- ❑ idursulfase
- ❑ Imuran
- ❑ Indocin
- ❑ Inflamase
- ❑ Infliximab
- ❑ Kenalog
- ❑ ketoprofen
- ❑ Kneerelief
- ❑ leflunomide
- ❑ Limbrel
- ❑ Liquid Pred
- ❑ Lodine
- ❑ Lopurin
- ❑ Medralone
- ❑ Medrol
- ❑ methotrexate
- ❑ methylprednisolone
- ❑ Mexate
- ❑ Mono-Gesic

ARTHRITIS

- ❏ Motrin
- ❏ Myochrysine
- ❏ Nalfon
- ❏ Neoral
- ❏ Naprelan
- ❏ Naprosyn
- ❏ naproxcinod
- ❏ naproxen
- ❏ Nuflexxa
- ❏ Orencia
- ❏ Orthovisc
- ❏ Orudis
- ❏ Oruvail
- ❏ Osteo Bi-Flex
- ❏ Pediapred
- ❏ penicillamine
- ❏ Pennsaid
- ❏ Pharma Flex
- ❏ piroxicam
- ❏ Plaqueril
- ❏ PN 400
- ❏ prednisolone
- ❏ prednisone
- ❏ Prelone
- ❏ probenecid
- ❏ Raptiva
- ❏ Reclast
- ❏ Relafen
- ❏ Remicade
- ❏ Rheumatrex
- ❏ Ridaura
- ❏ Rituxan
- ❏ rituximab
- ❏ rofecoxib
- ❏ Salonpas
- ❏ Satogesic
- ❏ Simponi
- ❏ sodium hyaluronate

ARTHRITIS

- ❏ Solu-Cortef
- ❏ Solu-Medrol
- ❏ sulfinpyrazone
- ❏ sulindac
- ❏ Supartz
- ❏ Synvisc
- ❏ Synvisc-One
- ❏ Thera-Gesic
- ❏ ThermaCare
- ❏ tocilizumab
- ❏ Tolectin
- ❏ tolmetin sodium
- ❏ Triam-A injection
- ❏ Tri-Kort
- ❏ Trilisate
- ❏ Trilog
- ❏ TripleFlex
- ❏ Trisoject injection
- ❏ valdecoxib
- ❏ Vimovo
- ❏ Vioxx
- ❏ Voltaren
- ❏ Zeel
- ❏ zoledronic acid
- ❏ Zyloprim

ASTHMA

- ❏ Accolate
- ❏ AccuNeb
- ❏ aclidinium bromide
- ❏ Advair Diskus
- ❏ Advair HFA
- ❏ Aerobid
- ❏ AeroCount
- ❏ Aerolate
- ❏ Airet

ASTHMA

- ❏ albuterol
- ❏ AllerNaze
- ❏ Allupent
- ❏ alpha1-proteinase
- ❏ alpha-proteinase
- ❏ Alvesco
- ❏ aminophylline
- ❏ Ana-Guard
- ❏ Anti-Ige
- ❏ Aralast NP
- ❏ Arcapta
- ❏ ardeparin sodium
- ❏ arformoterol tartrate
- ❏ Aridol
- ❏ Arm-A-Med
- ❏ Asmanex Twisthaler
- ❏ Astepro
- ❏ Asthmahaler
- ❏ Asthmalix
- ❏ AsthmaNefrin
- ❏ Atrovent
- ❏ azelastine
- ❏ Azmacort
- ❏ aztreonam lysine
- ❏ beclomethasone
- ❏ Beclovent
- ❏ bitolterol mesylate
- ❏ Brethaire
- ❏ Brethine
- ❏ Bricanyl
- ❏ Bronkaid
- ❏ Bronkephrine
- ❏ Bronkosol
- ❏ Brovana
- ❏ butesonide
- ❏ calcitriol
- ❏ Cayston
- ❏ ceftaroline fosamil
- ❏ Choledyl

ASTHMA

- ❏ ciclesonide
- ❏ Combivent
- ❏ cromolyn
- ❏ Daxas
- ❏ Daliresp
- ❏ Decadron Turbinaire
- ❏ Deltasone
- ❏ Dexacort
- ❏ Dey-Dose
- ❏ dexamethasone
- ❏ Dulera
- ❏ Duo-Inhaler
- ❏ DuoNeb
- ❏ dyphylline
- ❏ Elixophyllin-KI
- ❏ epinephrine
- ❏ Epi-Pen
- ❏ fenoterol
- ❏ Flonase
- ❏ Flo-Pred
- ❏ Flovent
- ❏ flunisolide
- ❏ fluticasone
- ❏ fluticasone furoate
- ❏ fluticasone propionate
- ❏ Flutiform
- ❏ Foradil Aerolizer
- ❏ formoterol fumarate
- ❏ Glassia
- ❏ guaifenesin
- ❏ Guai-Vent/PSE
- ❏ hylan
- ❏ indacaterol
- ❏ Intal Inhaler
- ❏ ipratropium bromide
- ❏ isoetharine
- ❏ isoproterenol
- ❏ Isuprel
- ❏ Lanophyllin

ASTHMA

- ❑ Levalbuterol
- ❑ levocetirizine dihydrochloride
- ❑ mannitol
- ❑ Maxair Autohaler
- ❑ Medaprel
- ❑ Medihaler
- ❑ Medrol
- ❑ Metaprel
- ❑ metaproterenol
- ❑ methylprednisolone
- ❑ mometasone furoate
- ❑ montelukast
- ❑ Motavizumab
- ❑ Nasacort AQ
- ❑ Nasalcrom
- ❑ Nasalide
- ❑ Nasonex
- ❑ nedocromil
- ❑ Novosalmol
- ❑ olopatadine
- ❑ omalizumab
- ❑ Orapred
- ❑ organidin
- ❑ oxtriphylline
- ❑ Patanase
- ❑ Pedipred
- ❑ Perforomist
- ❑ pirbuterol
- ❑ prednisolone
- ❑ prednisone
- ❑ Prelone
- ❑ Primatene Mist
- ❑ ProAir HFA
- ❑ Prolastin
- ❑ Proventil
- ❑ provocholine
- ❑ Pulmicort Respules
- ❑ Pulmicort Turbhaler

ASTHMA

- ❑ QAB149
- ❑ Quadrinal
- ❑ Quibron-T/SR
- ❑ QVAR
- ❑ Resogbud
- ❑ roflumilast
- ❑ salmeterol
- ❑ Serevent
- ❑ Singulair
- ❑ Slo-Bid
- ❑ Spiriva
- ❑ Spiriva HandiHaler
- ❑ Sus-Phrine
- ❑ Symbicort
- ❑ Teflaro
- ❑ terbutaline
- ❑ Theo-24
- ❑ Theochron
- ❑ Theo-Dur
- ❑ theophylline
- ❑ Tilade
- ❑ tiotropium bromide
- ❑ Tornalate
- ❑ triamcinolone
- ❑ turbutaline
- ❑ Uni-Dur
- ❑ Uniphyl
- ❑ Vanceril
- ❑ Ventolin
- ❑ Veramyst
- ❑ Volmax
- ❑ Xolair
- ❑ Xopenex
- ❑ Xyzal
- ❑ zafirlukast
- ❑ Zileuton
- ❑ Zyflo
- ❑ Zyflo CR

BIRTH CONTROL

- ❑ Alesse
- ❑ All-Flex diaphragm
- ❑ Apri
- ❑ Aviane
- ❑ Beyaz
- ❑ Brevicon
- ❑ BufferGel
- ❑ Conceptrol
- ❑ condom
- ❑ Copper 7
- ❑ Cryselle
- ❑ Cyclessa
- ❑ Dalkan Shield
- ❑ Delfen
- ❑ Demulen
- ❑ Depo-Provera
- ❑ Desogen
- ❑ desogestrel
- ❑ dienogest
- ❑ dinoprostone
- ❑ drospirenone
- ❑ ella
- ❑ EMKO
- ❑ Empresse
- ❑ Enovid
- ❑ Essure
- ❑ estradiol valerate
- ❑ Estrostep
- ❑ ethyl estradiol
- ❑ ethynodiol diacetate
- ❑ etonogestrel
- ❑ Fem-Cap
- ❑ Femcon FE
- ❑ Femhrt
- ❑ GenCept
- ❑ Genora
- ❑ Implanon
- ❑ Jadelle

BIRTH CONTROL

- ❑ Jenest
- ❑ Jolivette
- ❑ Kariva
- ❑ Koro-Flex
- ❑ Koromax
- ❑ KY-Plus
- ❑ Leena
- ❑ Levlen
- ❑ Levlite
- ❑ levomefolate
- ❑ levonorgestrel
- ❑ Levora
- ❑ Lippes Loop
- ❑ Loestrin
- ❑ Loestrin 24 Fe
- ❑ Lo Loestrin Fe
- ❑ Lo/Ovral
- ❑ LoSeasonique
- ❑ Low-Ogestrel
- ❑ Lunelle
- ❑ Lybrel
- ❑ Marvalon
- ❑ medroxyprogesterone
- ❑ mestranol
- ❑ Microgestin
- ❑ Micronor
- ❑ mifeprex
- ❑ mifepristone
- ❑ Ministrin
- ❑ Min-Ovral
- ❑ Mircette
- ❑ Mirena
- ❑ Modicon
- ❑ Mononessa
- ❑ Natazia
- ❑ Necon
- ❑ Nelova
- ❑ nonoxynol-9

BIRTH CONTROL

- ❑ Nora-BE
- ❑ Nordette
- ❑ norelgestromin
- ❑ Norethin
- ❑ norethindrone
- ❑ Norgestimate
- ❑ norgestrel
- ❑ Norinyl
- ❑ Norplant
- ❑ Nor-QD
- ❑ Nortrel
- ❑ NuvaRing
- ❑ Ocella
- ❑ Ogestrel
- ❑ Ortho-Cept
- ❑ Ortho-Creme
- ❑ Ortho-Cyclen
- ❑ Ortho-Evra
- ❑ Ortho-Gynol
- ❑ Ortho-Micronor
- ❑ Ortho-Novum
- ❑ Ortho-Prefest
- ❑ Ortho Tri-Cyclen
- ❑ Ortho Tri-Cyclen Lo
- ❑ Ovcon
- ❑ Ovral
- ❑ Ovrette
- ❑ ParaGard T280
- ❑ Plan B
- ❑ Portia
- ❑ Preven Emergency Kit
- ❑ Progestasert
- ❑ prostaglandine
- ❑ Prostin E2
- ❑ Qlaira
- ❑ Quasense
- ❑ Reclipsen
- ❑ RU-486

BIRTH CONTROL

- ❑ Safyral
- ❑ Seasonale
- ❑ Seasonique
- ❑ Select
- ❑ Semicid
- ❑ Solurex
- ❑ Sronyx
- ❑ Symphasic
- ❑ Tilia FE
- ❑ Tri-levlin
- ❑ TriNessa
- ❑ Tri-Norinyl
- ❑ Triphasil
- ❑ Triquilar
- ❑ Tri-Sprintec
- ❑ Trivora
- ❑ ulipristal acetate
- ❑ VasClip
- ❑ VCF Film
- ❑ WC 3016
- ❑ Yaz
- ❑ Yasmin
- ❑ ZenChent
- ❑ Zovia

BLEEDING DISORDERS

- ❑ albumin
- ❑ antithrombin
- ❑ ATryn
- ❑ BeneFIX
- ❑ BleedArrest
- ❑ Ceprotin
- ❑ Cera
- ❑ cyanocobalamin
- ❑ Cycrin
- ❑ Dacogen

BLEEDING DISORDERS

- ❑ DDAVP
- ❑ decitabine
- ❑ deferasirox
- ❑ eculizumab
- ❑ Evithrom
- ❑ Exjade
- ❑ Fibrinogen
- ❑ Flexbumin
- ❑ Helixate FS
- ❑ Humate-P
- ❑ Injectafer
- ❑ Kogenate
- ❑ Kuvan
- ❑ Methergine
- ❑ methoxy polyethylene glycol-epoetin
- ❑ methylergonovine
- ❑ Mircera
- ❑ Nascobal
- ❑ NovoSeven
- ❑ Privigen
- ❑ Provera
- ❑ Recothrom
- ❑ RiaSTAP
- ❑ sapropterin dihydrochloride
- ❑ Soliris
- ❑ Stimate
- ❑ Thrombin
- ❑ Thrombin-JMI
- ❑ Wilate
- ❑ Xyntha

CANCER

- ❑ abiraterone
- ❑ Abraxane
- ❑ Abstral
- ❑ ABVD

CANCER

- ❑ ABX-EGF
- ❑ AC
- ❑ ACe
- ❑ Actiq
- ❑ Adcetris
- ❑ Adriamycin
- ❑ Affinitak
- ❑ Afinitor
- ❑ albinterferon alfa-2b
- ❑ aldesleukin
- ❑ alemtuzumab
- ❑ Alimta
- ❑ Alkeran
- ❑ allopurinol
- ❑ Aloprim
- ❑ Aloxi
- ❑ altretamine
- ❑ Amen
- ❑ A-Methopterin
- ❑ amifostine
- ❑ anastrozole
- ❑ Android
- ❑ ANX-530
- ❑ Anzemet
- ❑ APC8015
- ❑ APF530
- ❑ Aranesp
- ❑ Aredia
- ❑ Arimidex
- ❑ Aromasin
- ❑ Arranon
- ❑ arsenic trioxide
- ❑ Arzerra
- ❑ asparaginase
- ❑ Avastin
- ❑ AVDP
- ❑ Avinza
- ❑ Avodart

CANCER

- ❑ axitinib
- ❑ azacitidine
- ❑ BACOP
- ❑ Baraclude
- ❑ bendamustine
- ❑ BEP
- ❑ bevacizumab
- ❑ bexarotene
- ❑ Bexxar
- ❑ bicalutamide
- ❑ BiCNU
- ❑ Blenoxane
- ❑ boceprevir
- ❑ bortezomib
- ❑ brentuximab vedotin
- ❑ Bryostatin
- ❑ Buserelin
- ❑ busulfan
- ❑ Busulfex
- ❑ cabazitaxel
- ❑ cabergoline
- ❑ CAF
- ❑ Campath
- ❑ Camptosar
- ❑ CAP
- ❑ capecitabine
- ❑ Caprelsa
- ❑ carboplatin
- ❑ Carbo-Tax
- ❑ carfilzomib
- ❑ carmustine
- ❑ Casamet
- ❑ Casodex
- ❑ CAVE
- ❑ CAV/VAC
- ❑ CC
- ❑ CCNU
- ❑ CD

CANCER

- ❑ CDDP/VP
- ❑ CDDP/VP-16
- ❑ CeeNu
- ❑ Ceplene
- ❑ Cera
- ❑ Cerubidine
- ❑ Cervarix
- ❑ cetuximab
- ❑ CFM
- ❑ CFPT
- ❑ chlorambucil
- ❑ Chl/VPP
- ❑ CHOP-Bleo
- ❑ CHOP
    - cyclophosphamide
    - doxorubicin
    - vincristine
    - prednisolone
- ❑ cinacalcet
- ❑ CISCA
- ❑ Cisplatin
- ❑ citarabine
- ❑ cladribine
- ❑ CLD-BOMP
- ❑ clofarabine
- ❑ Clolar
- ❑ clonidine
- ❑ CMF
- ❑ CMFP
- ❑ CMV
- ❑ CNOP
- ❑ COB
- ❑ COMLA
- ❑ COMP
- ❑ COP
- ❑ COP-BLAM
- ❑ COPE
- ❑ copegus

CANCER

- COPP
- Corzyme
- Cosmegen
- Cotara
- Cox-2 inhibitor
- CP
- crizotinib
- CT
- CVD
- CVD+IL 21
- CVP
- CVPP
- Cy/A
- cyclophosphamide
- Cysview
- Cytadren
- Cytosar
- Cytoxin
- CYVADIC
- DA
- dacarbazine
- dactinomycin
- dalteparin
- dasatinib
- DAT
- DAT/DCT
- daunomycin
- Daunorubicin
- DAV
- Degarelix
- denosumab
- Depo-Cyt
- Depo-Provera
- dexrazoxane
- DHAP
- DI
- Didronel
- Diflucan

CANCER

- DMC
- docetaxel
- Dolasetron
- Dostinex
- Doxil
- doxorubicin
- Drabinol
- Droxia
- DTIC-Dome
- Duraclon
- dutasteride
- EAP
- EC
- EDAP
- ELF
- Eligard
- Elitek
- Ellence
- Eloxatin
- Elspar
- EMA-86
- Emcyt
- Emend
- entecavir
- EPEG
- Epirubicin
- Epogen
- Epothilone
- EP/PE
- epratuzumab
- Erbitux
- Ergamisol
- eribulin mesylate
- erlotinib
- Erwinase
- ESHAP
- Estinyl
- estramustine

CANCER

- ❏ Estratab
- ❏ ET-743
- ❏ Ethyol
- ❏ Etopophos
- ❏ etoposide
- ❏ Eulexin
- ❏ EVA
- ❏ everolimus
- ❏ Evista
- ❏ Exelbine
- ❏ exemestane
- ❏ Exisulind
- ❏ FAC
- ❏ FAM
- ❏ FAME
- ❏ FAMTX
- ❏ Fareston
- ❏ Faslodex
- ❏ FCE
- ❏ F-CL
- ❏ fenofibric
- ❏ fentanyl citrate
- ❏ Fentora
- ❏ Feraheme
- ❏ ferumoxytol
- ❏ filgrastim
- ❏ Fle
- ❏ floxuridine
- ❏ Fludara
- ❏ fludarabine
- ❏ flutamide
- ❏ FMV
- ❏ Folotyn
- ❏ fosaprepitant dimeglumine
- ❏ Fragmin
- ❏ FUDR
- ❏ FU/LV
- ❏ fulvestrant

CANCER

- ❏ Fusilev
- ❏ Gardasil
- ❏ gemcitabine
- ❏ gemcitabine-Cis
- ❏ gemtuzumab
- ❏ Gemzar
- ❏ Genasense
- ❏ Gleevec
- ❏ Gliadel
- ❏ glucocerebrosidase
- ❏ goserelin
- ❏ granisetron
- ❏ Halaven
- ❏ HDMGTX
- ❏ HDMTX
- ❏ Hematide
- ❏ HepaGam B
- ❏ Herceptin
- ❏ Hexalen
- ❏ hexaminolevulinate
- ❏ Hexvix
- ❏ HI-CDAZE
- ❏ Hycamtin
- ❏ Hydrea
- ❏ hydroxurea
- ❏ ibritumomab tiuxetan
- ❏ ICE
- ❏ Idamycin
- ❏ idarubicin
- ❏ IDMTX/6-MP
- ❏ IE
- ❏ IFEX
- ❏ ifosfamide
- ❏ IFoVP
- ❏ imatinib
- ❏ IMF
- ❏ IMGN529
- ❏ IMVP-16

CANCER

- ❏ Incivek
- ❏ Infergen
- ❏ interferon
- ❏ interferon alfacon-1
- ❏ Intron A
- ❏ ipilimumab
- ❏ Iressa
- ❏ irinotecan
- ❏ Isovorin
- ❏ Istodax
- ❏ ixabepilone
- ❏ Ixempra
- ❏ Jevtana
- ❏ Kepivance
- ❏ Kytril
- ❏ lanreotide acetate
- ❏ lapatinib
- ❏ laromustine
- ❏ L-asparaginase
- ❏ Lanzanda
- ❏ LDAC
- ❏ lenalidomide
- ❏ Leucovorin
- ❏ Leukeran
- ❏ Leukine
- ❏ leuprolide
- ❏ Leustatin
- ❏ levoleucovorin
- ❏ Lexidronam
- ❏ livamisole
- ❏ Locteron
- ❏ lomustine
- ❏ Loramyc
- ❏ Lucassin
- ❏ Lupron
- ❏ L-VAM
- ❏ Lysodren
- ❏ MACOP-B

CANCER

- ❏ MAID
- ❏ Marinol
- ❏ Matulane
- ❏ m-BACOD
- ❏ M-BACOS
- ❏ MC
- ❏ mechlorethamine
- ❏ medroxyprogesterone
- ❏ Megace
- ❏ melphalan
- ❏ mercapturine
- ❏ mesna
- ❏ Mesnex
- ❏ methotrexate
- ❏ methyl aminolevulinate
- ❏ Metvixia
- ❏ micafungin
- ❏ miconazole lauriad
- ❏ MINE
- ❏ MINE-ESHAP
- ❏ Mithricin
- ❏ mitomycin
- ❏ mitoxantrone
- ❏ MM
- ❏ MMC
- ❏ MOBP
- ❏ MOP
- ❏ MOPP
- ❏ MOPP/ABV Hybrid
- ❏ MP
- ❏ m-PFL
- ❏ MTX
- ❏ MTX/6-MP
- ❏ MTX/6-MP/VP
- ❏ MTX-CDDPAdr
- ❏ Mustargen
- ❏ Mutamycin
- ❏ MV

CANCER

CANCER

- ❏ MVAC
- ❏ MVPP
- ❏ Mycamine
- ❏ Myleran
- ❏ Mylotarg
- ❏ Nabilone
- ❏ NasalFent
- ❏ Navelbine
- ❏ nelarabine
- ❏ Neovastat
- ❏ Neulasta
- ❏ Neupogen
- ❏ Nexavar
- ❏ NFL
- ❏ Nilandron
- ❏ nilotinib
- ❏ nilutamide
- ❏ Nipent
- ❏ Nolvadex
- ❏ Novantrone
- ❏ NOVP
- ❏ Noxafil
- ❏ Nplate
- ❏ Nuvion
- ❏ oblimersen
- ❏ octreotide
- ❏ ofatumumab
- ❏ omacetaxine mepesuccinate
- ❏ Omapro
- ❏ Oncaspar
- ❏ Oncolym
- ❏ Oncovin
- ❏ On-Q
- ❏ Onrigin
- ❏ Onsolis
- ❏ Ontak
- ❏ OPA
- ❏ OPPA

- ❏ OraVescent Fentanyl
- ❏ Orzel
- ❏ OvaRex
- ❏ oxaliplatin
- ❏ ozogamicin
- ❏ PAC
- ❏ paclitaxel
- ❏ palifermin
- ❏ pamidronate
- ❏ panitumumab
- ❏ papillomavirus
- ❏ Paraplatin
- ❏ pazopanib
- ❏ PC
- ❏ PCV
- ❏ pegaspargase
- ❏ pegfilgrastim
- ❏ peginterferon
- ❏ PEG-Intron
- ❏ pemetrexed
- ❏ PFL
- ❏ PFL+IFN
- ❏ Photofrin
- ❏ pilocarpine
- ❏ pixantrone
- ❏ Pixuvri
- ❏ placlitaxel
- ❏ Platinol
- ❏ Plenaxis
- ❏ plicamycin
- ❏ POC
- ❏ POMP
    - Purinethol
    - Oncovin
    - Methotrexate
    - Prednisone
- ❏ porfimer sodium
- ❏ posaconazole

CANCER

- ❏ pralatrexate
- ❏ prGCD
- ❏ Procrit
- ❏ Proleukin
- ❏ ProMACE-CytaBOM
- ❏ Provenge
- ❏ Pt-EU
- ❏ PTK 787
- ❏ Pt/VM
- ❏ Purinethol
- ❏ PVB
- ❏ PVD
- ❏ PVDA
- ❏ Quadramet
- ❏ quadrivalent
- ❏ Raloxifene
- ❏ Rapinyl
- ❏ rasburicase
- ❏ rebetol
- ❏ Revlimid
- ❏ ribasphere
- ❏ Ribavirin
- ❏ ridaforolimus
- ❏ Rituxan
- ❏ rituximab
- ❏ Roferon
- ❏ romidepsin
- ❏ romiplostim
- ❏ Rubex
- ❏ Ruxolitinib
- ❏ Salagen
- ❏ Sancuso
- ❏ Sandostatin
- ❏ sargramostim
- ❏ Sativex
- ❏ Sclerosol
- ❏ Sensipar
- ❏ Sequential Dox-CMF

CANCER

- ❏ sipuleucel-T
- ❏ SMF
- ❏ Soltamox
- ❏ Somatuline Autogel
- ❏ Somatuline Depot
- ❏ sorafenib
- ❏ Sprycel
- ❏ Stanford V
- ❏ streptozocin
- ❏ Sugen
- ❏ sunitinib
- ❏ Suprefact
- ❏ Sutent
- ❏ SU-101
- ❏ SU 11248
- ❏ Sylatron
- ❏ Tabloid
- ❏ Tamoxifen
- ❏ Tarceva
- ❏ Targretin
- ❏ Tasigna
- ❏ Taxol
- ❏ Taxotere
- ❏ telaprevir
- ❏ telbivudine
- ❏ Temodar
- ❏ temozolomide
- ❏ temsirolimus
- ❏ teniposide
- ❏ tenofovir disoproxil fumarate
- ❏ terlipressin
- ❏ Teslac
- ❏ testolactone
- ❏ Testred
- ❏ TheraCys
- ❏ ThermoDox
- ❏ thioguanine
- ❏ Thioplex

CANCER

- ❏ thiotepa
- ❏ Thyrogen
- ❏ ThyroShield
- ❏ TICE BCG
- ❏ TIP
- ❏ TIT
- ❏ Topo/CTX
- ❏ topotecan
- ❏ Toposar
- ❏ toremifene
- ❏ Torisel
- ❏ tositumomab
- ❏ Totect
- ❏ Trabectedin
- ❏ tranylcypromine sulfate
- ❏ trastuzumab
- ❏ Treanda
- ❏ Trelstar
- ❏ Trelstar LA
- ❏ tretinoin
- ❏ Trexall
- ❏ Trilipix
- ❏ triptorelin pamoate
- ❏ Trisenox
- ❏ Tykerb
- ❏ Tyzeka
- ❏ Uvadex
- ❏ VAB VI
- ❏ VAC
- ❏ VACAdr
- ❏ VACAdr-IfoVP
- ❏ VAD
- ❏ VAdrC
- ❏ Valstar
- ❏ Vancomycin
- ❏ vandetanib
- ❏ VATH
- ❏ VBAP
- ❏ VBMCP

CANCER

- ❏ VBP
- ❏ VCAP
- ❏ Vectibix
- ❏ velaglucerase alfa
- ❏ Velban
- ❏ Velcade
- ❏ vemurafenib
- ❏ VePesid
- ❏ Vesanoid
- ❏ Victrelis
- ❏ Vidaza
- ❏ vinblastine
- ❏ vincristine
- ❏ vinorelbine
- ❏ Vinorelbine-Cis
- ❏ VIP
- ❏ VIP [Einhorn]
- ❏ Viread
- ❏ Vismodegib
- ❏ vorinostat
- ❏ Votrient
- ❏ VP
- ❏ Vumon
- ❏ Xalkori
- ❏ Xcytrin
- ❏ Xeloda
- ❏ Yervoy
- ❏ Zactima
- ❏ Zalbin
- ❏ Zanosar
- ❏ Zelboraf
- ❏ Zevalin
- ❏ Zinecard
- ❏ Zofran
- ❏ Zoladex
- ❏ Zolinza
- ❏ Zyloprim
- ❏ Zytiga

CARDIOLOGY

- Abbokinase
- abciximab
- Accupril
- Accuretic
- Aceon
- ACOVA
- Activase
- Adalat
- Adcirca
- Adenocard
- Adenoscan
- adenosine
- Advicor
- Afeditab CR
- Aggrastat
- Aggrenox
- Agrylin
- Aldactazide
- Aldactone
- Aldoclor
- Aldomet
- Aldoril
- aliskiren
- Altace
- alteplase
- Altoprev
- ambrisentan
- amiloride
- Aminohippurate
- amiodarone
- amlodipine
- amlodipine besylate
- Amturnide
- Ana-Kit
- Ancrod
- Ancobon
- Angiomax
- Anhydron

CARDIOLOGY

- anisindione
- Antara
- ApoA-1
- ApoA-1 Milano
- aprotinin
- Aquatensen
- Aramine
- Aranesp
- Argatroban
- Arixtra
- Atacand
- Atenolol
- Atorvastatin
- Atromid-S
- Avalide
- Avapro
- azilsartan medoxomil
- Azor
- Baycol
- Benazepril
- bendroflumethiazide
- Benicar
- benzthiazide
- bepridil
- Betapace
- BiDil
- binodenoson
- bivalirudin
- Blocadren
- Brevibloc
- Brilinta
- bucindolol
- Bumetanide
- Bystolic
- Caduet
- Calan
- candesartan cilexetil
- Captopen

CARDIOLOGY

- ❏ Captopril
- ❏ Captozide
- ❏ Cardene
- ❏ Cardio Essentials
- ❏ CardioGen 82
- ❏ cardioplegic solution
- ❏ Cardioquin
- ❏ CardioTec Kit
- ❏ Cardizem
- ❏ Cardura
- ❏ Cartia XT
- ❏ Cartrol
- ❏ Carvedilol
- ❏ Catapres
- ❏ Catapres-TTS
- ❏ Cathflo Activase
- ❏ cerivastatin
- ❏ Certriad
- ❏ chlorothiazide
- ❏ chlorthalidone
- ❏ cholestyramine
- ❏ cilostazol
- ❏ clevidipine
- ❏ Cleviprex
- ❏ clofibrate
- ❏ clopidogrel
- ❏ Clorpres-TTS
- ❏ Colestid
- ❏ colestipol
- ❏ colesevelam
- ❏ Combipres
- ❏ Cordarone
- ❏ Coreg
- ❏ Coricidin HBP
- ❏ Corlopam
- ❏ Corvert
- ❏ CorVue
- ❏ Corzide

CARDIOLOGY

- ❏ Covera-HS
- ❏ Cozaar
- ❏ CP-529
- ❏ Crestor
- ❏ cyclothiazide
- ❏ dabigatran etexilate
- ❏ dalteparin
- ❏ danaparoid
- ❏ Daramode
- ❏ Daranide
- ❏ Darbepoetin Alfa
- ❏ Demadex
- ❏ Demser
- ❏ Deponit
- ❏ diatrizoate
- ❏ dibenzyline
- ❏ dichlorphenamide
- ❏ Digibind
- ❏ Digitek
- ❏ digoxin
- ❏ Dilacor XR
- ❏ Diltazem
- ❏ Diovan
- ❏ dipyridamole
- ❏ Diucardin
- ❏ Diuchlor
- ❏ Diulo
- ❏ Diupres
- ❏ Diuril
- ❏ dobutamine
- ❏ Dobutrex
- ❏ dofetilide
- ❏ Doxazosin
- ❏ dronedarone
- ❏ Durectic
- ❏ DX-88
- ❏ Dyazide
- ❏ Dyrenium

CARDIOLOGY

- ecallantide
- Ecotrin
- eculizumab
- Edarbi
- Edecrine
- Effient
- Eminase
- enalapril maleate
- Encainide
- Endeavor
- Enduron
- Enkaid
- enoxaparin
- Epi-Pen
- Epitope
- Epoprostenol
- eprosartan mesylate
- eptifibatide
- erythropoietin
- Esidrix
- Esimil
- esmolol
- ethacrynate sodium
- ethacrynic
- ethaverine
- Ethavex-100
- Ethmozine
- Exanta
- Exforge
- Exforge HCT
- Exna
- ezetimibe
- felodipine
- fenofibrate
- fenofibric
- Fenoglide
- flecainide
- Flolan

CARDIOLOGY

- flucytosine
- Fluidex
- fluvastatin
- fondaparinux
- Fragmin
- Furosemide
- gemfibrozil
- Genabid
- Gencaro
- Glucagon
- glucose
- Glutose
- glyceryl trinitrate
- Guanabenz
- Guanadrel
- Guanethidine
- guanfacine
- Halfprin
- Hespan
- hetastarch
- hydralazine hydrochloride
- Hydrex
- hydrochlorothiazide
- Hydro-D
- HydroDIURIL
- hydroflumethiazide
- Hydromox
- Hylorel
- Hyperstat
- Hytrin
- Hyzaar
- ibutilide
- Imdur
- Indapamide
- Inderal
- Inderide
- Innohep
- Integrilin

CARDIOLOGY

- Inversine
- irbesartan
- Ismelin
- ISMO
- Isoptin SR
- Isordil
- isosorbide dinitrate
- isoxsuprine
- Kabikinase
- Kalbitor
- Kerlone
- Kynapid
- Lanoxican
- Lanoxicaps
- Lanoxin
- Lasix
- lercanidipine
- Lescol
- Letairis
- Levatol
- Levostatin
- Lexiscan
- Lexxel
- Lipitor
- Livalo
- LoCholest
- Lofibra
- Lopid
- Lorelco
- losartan
- Lotrel
- lovastatin
- Lovaza
- Lovenox
- Mavik
- Maxzide
- Metahydrin
- methyclothiazide

CARDIOLOGY

- metolazone
- metoprolol
- Mevacor
- Mexitil
- Micardis
- micronized colestipol
- Microzide
- Midamor
- midodrine
- milrinone
- Minipress
- Minizide
- Mipomersen
- Moduretic
- Monoket
- Monopril
- moricizine
- Multaq
- Mykrox
- Nadolol
- Natrecor
- nebivolol
- Neo-Codema
- nesiritide
- Nexterone
- niacin
- Niaspan
- nicardipine
- Nicolar
- nifedipine
- nimodipine
- Nimotop
- Nisoldipine
- Nitro-Bid
- Nitro-Derm
- Nitrodisc
- Nitro-Dur
- nitroglycerin

CARDIOLOGY

- ❏ Nitrolingual
- ❏ NitroMist
- ❏ Nitrostat
- ❏ Normiflo
- ❏ Normodyne
- ❏ Norpace
- ❏ Norvasc
- ❏ Novo-Hydrazide
- ❏ Novo-Thalidone
- ❏ Odrinil
- ❏ olmesartan
- ❏ olmesartan medoxomil
- ❏ Omacor
- ❏ Oretic
- ❏ Orgaran
- ❏ Pacerone
- ❏ papaverine
- ❏ Pavabid
- ❏ Pavatine
- ❏ pentoxifylline
- ❏ Persantine
- ❏ phenylephrine
- ❏ phytosterol blocker
- ❏ pitavastatin
- ❏ Plavix
- ❏ Plegisol
- ❏ Plendil
- ❏ Pletal
- ❏ polythiazide
- ❏ Posicor
- ❏ Pradaxa
- ❏ prasugrel
- ❏ Pravachol
- ❏ pravastatin
- ❏ Pravigard
- ❏ Primacor
- ❏ Prinivil
- ❏ ProAmatine

CARDIOLOGY

- ❏ procainamide
- ❏ Procanbid
- ❏ Procardia
- ❏ Procrit Epoetin Alfa
- ❏ Proflavanol
- ❏ propafenone
- ❏ propranolol
- ❏ Prostin VR
- ❏ protamine sulfate
- ❏ Questran
- ❏ quinethazone
- ❏ Quin-G
- ❏ Quinidex
- ❏ quinidine
- ❏ Quin-Release
- ❏ Ranexa
- ❏ ranolazine
- ❏ Rasilez
- ❏ regadenoson
- ❏ Remodulin
- ❏ Renese
- ❏ ReoPro
- ❏ RESPeRATE
- ❏ Retavase
- ❏ Reteplase
- ❏ Revatio
- ❏ rosuvastatin
- ❏ Rythmol
- ❏ Saluron
- ❏ Sectral
- ❏ Ser-Ap-Es
- ❏ sildenafil citrate
- ❏ Simcor
- ❏ simvastatin
- ❏ sodium edecrin
- ❏ sodium nitroprusside
- ❏ Soliris
- ❏ Sorbitrate

CARDIOLOGY

- ❑ sotalol
- ❑ spironolactone
- ❑ stanozolol
- ❑ Streptase
- ❑ Streptokinase
- ❑ Sular
- ❑ Sunril
- ❑ tadalafil
- ❑ Tamocor
- ❑ Tarka
- ❑ Teczem
- ❑ Tekamlo
- ❑ Tekturna
- ❑ Tekturna HCT
- ❑ telmisartan
- ❑ tenecteplase
- ❑ Tenex
- ❑ Tenoretic
- ❑ Tenormin
- ❑ Teveten
- ❑ Thalitone
- ❑ Tiazac
- ❑ ticagrelor
- ❑ Ticlid
- ❑ ticlopidine
- ❑ Tikosyn
- ❑ Tilosyn
- ❑ tinzaparin
- ❑ tirofaban
- ❑ TNKase
- ❑ tocainide
- ❑ Tonocard
- ❑ Toprol-XL
- ❑ torcetrapib
- ❑ torsemide
- ❑ TPA
- ❑ trandolapril
- ❑ Trasylol

CARDIOLOGY

- ❑ Trental
- ❑ treprostinil
- ❑ triamterene
- ❑ Tribenzor
- ❑ trichlormethiazide
- ❑ TriCor
- ❑ Triglide
- ❑ Trilipix
- ❑ Twynsta
- ❑ Tyvaso
- ❑ UK-68-798
- ❑ Unvasc
- ❑ Uniretic
- ❑ Uridon
- ❑ Urozide
- ❑ valsartan
- ❑ Valturna
- ❑ Vanlev
- ❑ Vascor
- ❑ Vaseretic
- ❑ Vasodilan
- ❑ Vasotec
- ❑ Vasoxyl
- ❑ Ventavis
- ❑ verapamil
- ❑ Verelan
- ❑ vernakalant
- ❑ Vytorin
- ❑ Welchol
- ❑ Winstrol
- ❑ Wytensin
- ❑ Xience
- ❑ ximelagatran
- ❑ Zaroxolyn
- ❑ Zebeta
- ❑ Zestoretic
- ❑ Zestril
- ❑ Zetia

CARDIOLOGY

- ❏ Ziac
- ❏ Zinecard
- ❏ Zocor
- ❏ Zotarolimus

COLD+COUGH

- ❏ acetaminophen
- ❏ Acetavance
- ❏ Actifed
- ❏ Advil
- ❏ Alacor DM Syrup
- ❏ Afrin
- ❏ Alavert
- ❏ Alfa CF
- ❏ Allegra
- ❏ Allegra-D
- ❏ AllerNaze
- ❏ Allerx
- ❏ Allfen
- ❏ Aleve
- ❏ Aleve-D
- ❏ Alka-Seltzer Plus
- ❏ Ambifed
- ❏ Amerifed
- ❏ Anatuss
- ❏ Arco-Lase
- ❏ Ascriptin
- ❏ astemizole
- ❏ Astepro
- ❏ Atrohist
- ❏ Avelox
- ❏ Ayr
- ❏ azelastine
- ❏ Balamine
- ❏ Baltussin
- ❏ BDP Nasal

COLD+COUGH

- ❏ Benadryl
- ❏ Benadryl-D
- ❏ Benzedrex
- ❏ benzonatate
- ❏ Boiron
- ❏ Boostrix
- ❏ Boroleum
- ❏ Breathe Right
- ❏ Bromfed
- ❏ brompheniramine
- ❏ Brontex
- ❏ Bufferin
- ❏ Cantil
- ❏ cetirizine
- ❏ Cheracol
- ❏ Chloraseptic
- ❏ chlorpheniramine
- ❏ chlorpheniramine polistirex
- ❏ Chlor-Trimeton
- ❏ ciclesonide
- ❏ Clarinex
- ❏ Clarinex-D
- ❏ Claritin
- ❏ Claritin-D
- ❏ Codeprex
- ❏ Codiclear
- ❏ Coldcalm
- ❏ Cold-EEZE
- ❏ Comhist
- ❏ Comtrex
- ❏ Congess
- ❏ Contac
- ❏ Contac Cold + Flu
- ❏ Contac-D
- ❏ Contrave
- ❏ Coricidin
- ❏ Coricidin HBP
- ❏ Creomulsion

COLD+COUGH

- Cromolyn
- DayQuil
- Decacort
- Deconamine
- Deconsal
- Deconsat
- Delsym
- Desloratadine
- Despec
- dexamethasone
- dexbrompheniramine
- dextromethorphan
- Diabe-Tuss DM
- Diabetic Tussin
- Dimetane
- Dimetapp
- Diphedryl
- Dristan
- Drixoral
- Duratex
- Duratuss
- Echinacea
- Emergen-C
- Entex
- ENTSOL
- Excedrin
- Exgest
- Extendryl
- Fedahist
- fexofenadine
- glyceryl guaiacolate
- Guaifed
- guaifenesin
- Guaimax
- Halotussin
- Hismanal
- Histussin
- Humibid

COLD+COUGH

- hydrocodone
- Inspire
- Isoclor
- Kophane
- Kwelcof
- Liquibid
- Lufyllin
- Maxidone
- Mentholatum
- moxifloxacin
- Mucinex
- Mucinex D
- Mucinex DM
- Mucinex Mini-Melts
- Nasacort AQ
- NasalCrom
- Nasonex
- Neo-Synephrine
- Nostrilla
- NyQuil
- Nytol
- Ocean
- olopatadine
- Omnaris
- Oscillo
- Oscillococcinum
- Organidin
- Ornex
- Otrivin
- oxymetazoline
- Patanase
- PediaCare
- Pediacof
- Pedialyte
- Phenergan
- phenylephrine
- Picovir
- pleconaril

141

COLD+COUGH

- Profen IB
- Prometh
- promethazine
- Propel Implant
- pseudoephedrine
- Quadrinal
- Quenalin
- Quibron
- Quintex
- Rescon
- Rezira
- Rhinosyn
- Ricola
- Robitussin
- Robitussin CF
- Robitussin DAC
- Robitussin DM
- Robitussin DM Max
- Rondec
- Rynatan
- Rynatuss
- Sambucol
- Similasan
- Sine-Off
- Sinex
- SinoFresh
- SinuCleanse
- Sinulin
- Sinupan
- Sinutab
- Sominex
- Sudafed
- Sudafed OM
- Syn-Rx
- Tessalon
- Theraflu
- triamcinolone
- Triaminic

COLD+COUGH

- Triaminic Softchews
- Triaminicin
- Trinalin
- Tussagesic
- Tussend
- Tussin
- Tussionex Pennkinetic
- Tussi-Organindin DM
- Unisom
- VapoInhaler
- VapRub
- VapoSpray
- VapoSteam
- VapoSyrup
- VaporPatch
- Vicks
- Vicks 44D
- Vicks 44E
- Vicks Casero
- Vicks DayQuil
- Vicks NyQuil
- Vicks Sinex
- Vicks VapoRub
- Vicks VapoSteam
- West-Decon
- Westrim
- XL-3
- xylometazoline
- Zicam
- Zutripro
- Zyrtec
- Zyrtec D

DERMATOLOGY

- 8-Mop
- A+D

DERMATOLOGY

- Abreva
- Acanya
- Accutane
- acitretin
- Aclovate
- AcneFree
- Acthar Gel
- Acticin
- Actinex
- Actiza
- Aclovate
- ActiFade
- acyclovir
- Aczone
- adapalene
- Aftate
- Alba
- Albolene
- Alferon
- Aldara
- alitretinoin
- allium cepa
- Alpha-Hydroxy
- Altabax
- Alti-Acyclovir
- Alustra
- Ambi
- amcinonide
- Amevive
- aminolevulinic acid
- aminophylline
- AmLactin AP
- AmLactin XL
- Anbesol
- anidulafungin
- anthralin
- Anxanil
- Appearex

DERMATOLOGY

- Aquanil
- Aquaphor
- Aristocort
- Aristospan
- Artecoll
- Artefill
- Artiss
- Atrac-Tain
- Atarax
- Atopiclair
- Atralin
- A/T/S
- Australian Gold
- Avage
- Avalon Organics
- AVC
- Aveeno
- Avirax
- Avita
- Avobenzone
- azelaic acid
- azficel-T
- Azelex
- Azfibrocel-T
- bacitracin
- Bacitraycin
- Bactine
- Bain de Soleil
- Balmex
- Banana Boat
- Band-Aid Scar Healing
- Barbasol
- Belotero Balance
- Benadryl
- Benadryl-D
- Benoquin
- bentoquatam
- Benzac

143

DERMATOLOGY

- ❑ Benzaclin
- ❑ Benzamycin
- ❑ Benziq
- ❑ benzoyl peroxide
- ❑ benzyl alcohol
- ❑ Berinert
- ❑ betamethasone
- ❑ betamethasone dipropionate
- ❑ betamethasone valerate
- ❑ Beyaz
- ❑ bichloracetic acid Kahlenberg
- ❑ Biore
- ❑ Blistex
- ❑ Botox
- ❑ Brevoxyl
- ❑ Bull Frog
- ❑ Burt's Bees
- ❑ butenafine
- ❑ C1-esterase inhibitor
- ❑ Caladryl
- ❑ CalaGel
- ❑ Calahist
- ❑ calamine
- ❑ calcipotriene
- ❑ calcitriol
- ❑ Caldesene
- ❑ Campho-Phenique
- ❑ Capex
- ❑ capryloyl glycine
- ❑ Captique
- ❑ Carac cream
- ❑ Carlesta
- ❑ Carmex
- ❑ ceftaroline fosamil
- ❑ Cellulean
- ❑ CeraVe
- ❑ Cetaphil lotion
- ❑ ChapStick

DERMATOLOGY

- ❑ Cica-Care
- ❑ ciclopirox olamine
- ❑ Cinryze
- ❑ Claripel
- ❑ Clean & Clear
- ❑ Clearasil
- ❑ Clear Away
- ❑ Clenia
- ❑ Cleocin
- ❑ Clinac
- ❑ Clindagel
- ❑ clindamycin
- ❑ clindamycin hydrochloride
- ❑ Clioquinol
- ❑ clobetasol propionate
- ❑ Clobevate
- ❑ Clobex
- ❑ clotrimazole
- ❑ Collagenase
- ❑ Compound W
- ❑ Condylox
- ❑ Coppertone
- ❑ Cordran
- ❑ Cormax
- ❑ Cortaid
- ❑ corticotropin
- ❑ cortisone
- ❑ Cortisporin
- ❑ Cortone
- ❑ Cortizone-10
- ❑ CosmoDerm
- ❑ CosmoPlast
- ❑ cromolyn sodium
- ❑ crotamiton
- ❑ Curad Scar Therapy
- ❑ Curel
- ❑ Cutivate
- ❑ Cyclocort

DERMATOLOGY

- ❑ cyclosporine
- ❑ Dagenan
- ❑ dapsone
- ❑ Decaspray
- ❑ Denavir
- ❑ Denorex
- ❑ Dermaplast
- ❑ Dermarest
- ❑ DermaSmoothe
- ❑ Dermatop
- ❑ Desenex
- ❑ Desitin
- ❑ Desonate
- ❑ desonide
- ❑ Desowen
- ❑ desoxymetasone
- ❑ Desquam
- ❑ dexamethasone
- ❑ DHS tar shampoo
- ❑ Diabet-X
- ❑ Differin
- ❑ diflorasone
- ❑ Diprolene
- ❑ Diprosone
- ❑ Dithrocreme
- ❑ Dr. Scholl's
- ❑ Domeboro
- ❑ Dovonex
- ❑ doxepin
- ❑ drospirenone
- ❑ Duac
- ❑ DuoFilm
- ❑ Dysport
- ❑ efalizumab
- ❑ Eldopaque
- ❑ Eldoquin
- ❑ Eletone cream
- ❑ Elevess

DERMATOLOGY

- ❑ Elidel
- ❑ Elimite
- ❑ Elocon
- ❑ Emgel
- ❑ Enydrial
- ❑ Epiduo
- ❑ Ertaczo
- ❑ Erycette
- ❑ Erythra-Derm
- ❑ erythromycin ethylsuccinate
- ❑ esterase
- ❑ Estrostep
- ❑ ethyl
- ❑ ethyl estradiol
- ❑ ETS-2 %
- ❑ Eucerin
- ❑ Eurex
- ❑ Evoclin
- ❑ Evolence
- ❑ Excelderm
- ❑ Extina
- ❑ fibrin sealant
- ❑ Finacea
- ❑ Finevin
- ❑ Firazyr
- ❑ Flexitol
- ❑ Flexitol Blistop
- ❑ fluocinolone
- ❑ Fluoroplex
- ❑ fluorouracil
- ❑ fluticasone
- ❑ Formadon
- ❑ formaldehyde
- ❑ Fototar
- ❑ Fulvicin
- ❑ FungiCare
- ❑ FungiClear
- ❑ FungiCure

DERMATOLOGY

- ❑ Fungizone
- ❑ Fusion
- ❑ Garamycin
- ❑ Garnier
- ❑ Gillette
- ❑ glycerin
- ❑ glycyrrhetinic acid
- ❑ Glyquin
- ❑ Gold Bond
- ❑ Granulex
- ❑ Grifulvin
- ❑ griseofulvin
- ❑ GRIS-PEG
- ❑ halcinonide
- ❑ halobetasol
- ❑ Halog
- ❑ Hawaiian Tropic
- ❑ Head & Shoulders
- ❑ Herpecin-L
- ❑ Hibiclens
- ❑ Hibistat
- ❑ hydrocortisone
- ❑ Hydrocortone
- ❑ hydroquinone
- ❑ Hydroxatone
- ❑ hydroxyzine pamoate
- ❑ Hylaform
- ❑ hyaluronic acid
- ❑ Hytone
- ❑ icatibant
- ❑ Iclaprim
- ❑ imidazole
- ❑ imiquimod
- ❑ Impruv
- ❑ Instat
- ❑ interferon alfa
- ❑ Invanz
- ❑ iodoquinol

DERMATOLOGY

- ❑ Ionil-T
- ❑ Iontophoretic
- ❑ isopropyl
- ❑ isotretinoin
- ❑ Itch-X
- ❑ Ivarest
- ❑ IvyBLock
- ❑ Ivy-Dry
- ❑ IvyStat!
- ❑ Jason
- ❑ Jergens
- ❑ Juvederm
- ❑ Kank-A
- ❑ Kerastick
- ❑ Keralyt
- ❑ ketoconazole
- ❑ Klaron
- ❑ KP Duty
- ❑ kunecatechins
- ❑ L.M.X.4 cream
- ❑ L.M.X.5 cream
- ❑ Lac-Hydrin
- ❑ Laclotion
- ❑ Lamisil
- ❑ Lanacane
- ❑ lanolin
- ❑ laViv
- ❑ Lazerformaldehyde
- ❑ levocetirizine dihydrochloride
- ❑ levomefolate
- ❑ Levulan Kerastick
- ❑ Lidex
- ❑ LidoSite
- ❑ Lindane lotion
- ❑ Lipsovir
- ❑ Loprox
- ❑ L'OREAL
- ❑ Lotrimin

DERMATOLOGY

- ❑ Lotrisone
- ❑ Lubriderm
- ❑ Lumene
- ❑ Lustro
- ❑ Luxiq
- ❑ Malathion
- ❑ Masoprocol
- ❑ Maxiflor
- ❑ Mederma
- ❑ Melanax
- ❑ meloxicam
- ❑ Mentadil
- ❑ Mentax
- ❑ Merlot
- ❑ methoxsalen
- ❑ methyl aminolevulinate
- ❑ Metrocream
- ❑ Metrogel
- ❑ metronidazole cream
- ❑ Metvixia
- ❑ Micanol
- ❑ Micatin
- ❑ miconazole
- ❑ Mimyx
- ❑ Mintezol
- ❑ Miracle of Aloe Miracure
- ❑ Miranel
- ❑ Mobic
- ❑ Mobisyl
- ❑ Moisturel
- ❑ mometasone
- ❑ Monistat-Derm
- ❑ monobenzone
- ❑ Multipax
- ❑ Mycostatin
- ❑ Nads
- ❑ naftifine
- ❑ Naftin

DERMATOLOGY

- ❑ Nair
- ❑ Natroba
- ❑ Neoral
- ❑ Neosporin
- ❑ Neutrogena
- ❑ Nicomide
- ❑ nicotinamide
- ❑ Nivea
- ❑ Nix Crème
- ❑ Nizoral A-D
- ❑ Noah's Naturals
- ❑ NonyX
- ❑ Noritate
- ❑ Novitra
- ❑ Novo-Hydroxyzin
- ❑ Noxzema
- ❑ NuFill
- ❑ Nystatin
- ❑ Occusal-HP
- ❑ Olay
- ❑ Olay Regenerist
- ❑ Olux Foam
- ❑ Olux-E Foam
- ❑ onabotulinumtoxinA
- ❑ Orabase
- ❑ Oracea
- ❑ Orajel
- ❑ Ovide
- ❑ Oxistat
- ❑ Oxsoralen-Ultra
- ❑ Oxy
- ❑ Oxyconazole
- ❑ Paddock Podifilox
- ❑ Panafil
- ❑ Panafil SE
- ❑ Pandel
- ❑ PanOxyl
- ❑ Panretin gel

DERMATOLOGY

- ❏ penciclovir
- ❏ Perlabella
- ❏ Perlane
- ❏ pHisoderm
- ❏ pHisoHex
- ❏ pimecorlimus
- ❏ Pin-Rid
- ❏ Prelone
- ❏ Podocon
- ❏ podofilox
- ❏ Polyphenon E
- ❏ Polysporin
- ❏ Polytar shampoo
- ❏ Pond's
- ❏ Pramegel
- ❏ Pramosone
- ❏ prednisolone
- ❏ Preparation H
- ❏ Pro Clearz
- ❏ Prograniq
- ❏ Pronto
- ❏ Prosacea
- ❏ ProVectin
- ❏ Prudoxin
- ❏ Psorcon cream
- ❏ Psoriasin
- ❏ Purpose
- ❏ pyrantel pamoate
- ❏ Radiance
- ❏ Radiesse
- ❏ Raptiva
- ❏ Releev
- ❏ Renova
- ❏ Restylane
- ❏ retapamulin
- ❏ Retina-A-Micro
- ❏ Revitalift
- ❏ Rhucin

DERMATOLOGY

- ❏ Rid Lice
- ❏ Roc
- ❏ Rosac wash
- ❏ Safe 4 Hours
- ❏ St. Ives
- ❏ Salac
- ❏ salicylic acid
- ❏ Santyl
- ❏ Sarna
- ❏ Scalpicin
- ❏ Scar Away
- ❏ Scarguard
- ❏ Schick
- ❏ Sclerosol intrapleural
- ❏ Sculptra
- ❏ Sebazole
- ❏ Sebulex
- ❏ Selsun
- ❏ SERPACWA
- ❏ sertaconazole
- ❏ shea butter
- ❏ skinMilk
- ❏ Skintimate
- ❏ sodium sulfacetamide
- ❏ Solage
- ❏ Solarcaine
- ❏ Solodyn
- ❏ Soriatane
- ❏ Sorilux
- ❏ Spenco 2nd Skin Scar
- ❏ spinosad
- ❏ StaphAseptic
- ❏ Stelara
- ❏ Stridex
- ❏ StriVectin-HS
- ❏ StriVectin-SD
- ❏ sulconazole
- ❏ Sulfacet

DERMATOLOGY

- ❑ sulfapyridine
- ❑ Swabplus
- ❑ Synalar
- ❑ Synemol
- ❑ Synovium
- ❑ Taclonex
- ❑ Tanac
- ❑ Tavist
- ❑ tazarotene gel
- ❑ Tazorac
- ❑ Tecnu
- ❑ Teflaro
- ❑ telavancin
- ❑ Temovate
- ❑ terbinafine
- ❑ thalidomide
- ❑ Thalomid
- ❑ Thermage
- ❑ Thiobendazole
- ❑ tigecycline
- ❑ Tinactin
- ❑ Tinamed
- ❑ Tineacide
- ❑ tolnaftate
- ❑ Topicort
- ❑ tretinoin
- ❑ triamcinolone
- ❑ Triaz
- ❑ TriDerma
- ❑ Tridesilon
- ❑ Tri-Luma
- ❑ trioxsalen
- ❑ Trisoralen
- ❑ T-Stat
- ❑ Tucks
- ❑ Tygacil
- ❑ Ulesfia
- ❑ ULTRACEPT

DERMATOLOGY

- ❑ Ultravate
- ❑ Undelenic
- ❑ Uracil
- ❑ ustekinumab
- ❑ valacyclovir
- ❑ Valtrex
- ❑ Vanicream
- ❑ Vanos
- ❑ Vanoxide-HC lotion
- ❑ Vaseline
- ❑ Vectical
- ❑ Veet
- ❑ Velac
- ❑ Veltin
- ❑ Verdeso
- ❑ Veregen
- ❑ Vibativ
- ❑ Vioform
- ❑ Vistaril
- ❑ Vytone cream
- ❑ Water-Jel
- ❑ Westcort
- ❑ Woun-dres
- ❑ Xanelim
- ❑ Xenaderm
- ❑ Xolegel
- ❑ X-Seb T Plus
- ❑ Xyzal
- ❑ Yaz
- ❑ Yes to Carrots
- ❑ Yes to Cucumbers
- ❑ Yes to Tomatoes
- ❑ Zanfel
- ❑ ZAPZYT
- ❑ Zeasorb
- ❑ Zeasorb-AF
- ❑ Zetar Emulsion
- ❑ Ziana

DERMATOLOGY

- ❏ Zincon
- ❏ Zilactin
- ❏ Zonalon
- ❏ Zyclara
- ❏ ZymaDerm

DIABETES

- ❏ acarbose
- ❏ acetohexamide
- ❏ ACTOplus met
- ❏ Actos
- ❏ Afresa
- ❏ Afrezza
- ❏ alogliptin
- ❏ Amaryl
- ❏ Apidra
- ❏ Ascensia Breeze
- ❏ Aspart
- ❏ atorvastatin
- ❏ Avandaryl
- ❏ Avandia
- ❏ Breeze2
- ❏ bromocriptine mesylate
- ❏ Bydureon
- ❏ Byetta
- ❏ Ceftobiprole
- ❏ chlorpropamide
- ❏ colesevelam
- ❏ Cycloset
- ❏ Cymbalta
- ❏ Dapagliflozin
- ❏ DDAVP
- ❏ detemir
- ❏ DiaBeta
- ❏ Diabinese
- ❏ Diazoxide

DIABETES

- ❏ Duetact
- ❏ duloxetine
- ❏ Euglucon
- ❏ exenatide
- ❏ exendin-4
- ❏ Exubera
- ❏ Fortamet
- ❏ Gen-Glybe
- ❏ Glargine
- ❏ glimepiride
- ❏ glipizide
- ❏ Glucagen
- ❏ Glucagon
- ❏ Glucamide
- ❏ Glucophage
- ❏ Glucotrol
- ❏ Glucovance
- ❏ glulisine
- ❏ Glumetza
- ❏ glyburide
- ❏ Glynase
- ❏ Glynase Prestab
- ❏ Glyset
- ❏ Humalog Kwikpen
- ❏ Humalog Pen
- ❏ Humulin 50/50
- ❏ Humulin 70/30
- ❏ Humulin N
- ❏ Humulin R
- ❏ Iletin II, Lente
- ❏ Iletin Ii, NPH
- ❏ Iluvien
- ❏ Increlex
- ❏ Insulatard
- ❏ insulin
- ❏ insulin aspart protamine
- ❏ insulin detemir

DIABETES

- insulin glargine
- insulin glulisine
- insulin human
- insulin lispro
- insulin lispro protamine
- iPlex
- Janumet
- Januvia
- Juvisync
- Kombiglyze
- Lantus
- Lantus SoloStar
- Lente
- Lente Iletin II
- Levemir
- linagliptin
- Linjeta
- Lipitor
- liraglutide
- Lispro
- Lyrica
- mecasermin
- Medi-Glybe
- meglitinide
- metformin
- Metreleptin
- Micronase
- miglitol
- Mixtard
- Nataglinide
- Novo-Butamide
- Novo-Glyburide
- Novolin
- Novolin N PenFill
- NovolinPen
- NovoLog
- NovoPen

DIABETES

- NPH Iletin
- NPH Pork Isophane
- Nu-Glyburide
- Onglyza
- Orinase
- pioglitazone
- pramlintide
- PrandiMet
- Prandin
- Precose
- pregabalin
- Proglycem
- protamine zinc
- PZI
- Rezulin
- repaglinide
- rosiglitazone
- saxagliptin
- Semilente Iletin
- simvastatin
- sitagliptin
- SomatoKine
- Starlix
- sulfonylurea
- Symlin
- SYR-322
- Tolamide
- tolazamide
- tolbutamide
- Tolinase
- Tradjenta
- Ultralente
- Troglitazone
- Velosulin
- VIAject
- Victoza
- Welchol

DIGESTION

- ❑ Accuflora
- ❑ Align
- ❑ Alinia
- ❑ alosetron
- ❑ alpha-galactosidase
- ❑ Amitiza
- ❑ Beano
- ❑ Beano Meltaways
- ❑ Benefiber
- ❑ cantil
- ❑ Charcocaps
- ❑ Citrucel
- ❑ clindamycin
- ❑ Clindet
- ❑ Colase
- ❑ Colon Health
- ❑ Colonaide
- ❑ Coly-Mycin
- ❑ Culturelle
- ❑ Dexilant
- ❑ Dia-Quel
- ❑ Diastay
- ❑ Diastop
- ❑ difenoxin
- ❑ Donnagel
- ❑ Dulcolax
- ❑ Equalactin
- ❑ Evercleanse
- ❑ Ex-Lax
- ❑ Fiber Choice
- ❑ FiberCon
- ❑ Florastor
- ❑ furazolidone
- ❑ Furoxone
- ❑ Gas-X
- ❑ Gattex
- ❑ Homapin
- ❑ Imodium

DIGESTION

- ❑ Imodium A-D
- ❑ Kaolin
- ❑ Kao-Paverin
- ❑ Kaopectate
- ❑ Kasof
- ❑ Konsyl
- ❑ Lactaid
- ❑ Lactinex
- ❑ Linaclotide
- ❑ Little Tummys
- ❑ Liprotamase
- ❑ Lomotil
- ❑ loperamide
- ❑ Lotronex
- ❑ lubiprostone
- ❑ Metamucil
- ❑ Milk of Bismuth
- ❑ MiraLAX
- ❑ Motofen
- ❑ Mycifradin
- ❑ nitazoxanide
- ❑ Palsorb
- ❑ Paocin
- ❑ Paragel
- ❑ Paralixer
- ❑ Parepectolin
- ❑ Pectocel
- ❑ Pepto-Bismol
- ❑ Perdiem
- ❑ Phillips Milk of Magnesia
- ❑ probiotic
- ❑ Prunelax
- ❑ rifaximin
- ❑ Rotarix
- ❑ Rotateq
- ❑ rotavirus
- ❑ Senokot
- ❑ Senokot-S

DIGESTION

- ❏ SenokotXTRA
- ❏ Sustenex
- ❏ Swiss Kriss
- ❏ Xifaxan

FERTILITY

- ❏ anti-phospholipids
- ❏ A.P.L.
- ❏ apomorphine
- ❏ ArginMax
- ❏ Avimil
- ❏ Bravelle
- ❏ Bromocriptine
- ❏ cabergoline
- ❏ Cervidil
- ❏ Cetrorelix
- ❏ Cetrotide
- ❏ Chorex
- ❏ choriogonadotropin alfa
- ❏ chorionic gonadotropin
- ❏ Choron
- ❏ Cialis
- ❏ Clomid
- ❏ clomiphene citrate
- ❏ Corgonject
- ❏ Crinone
- ❏ Delestrogen
- ❏ Dostinex
- ❏ Edex
- ❏ Endometrin
- ❏ Fertinex
- ❏ Follistim
- ❏ Follistim/Antagon Kit
- ❏ follitropin alfa/beta
- ❏ Follutein
- ❏ Glukor

FERTILITY

- ❏ Gonadorelin
- ❏ Gonal
- ❏ Gonic
- ❏ Humegon
- ❏ Interex
- ❏ Levitra
- ❏ Livial
- ❏ Lutrepulse
- ❏ menotropin
- ❏ Metrodin
- ❏ Muse
- ❏ Novarel
- ❏ Ovidrel
- ❏ Parlodel
- ❏ Pergonal
- ❏ phentolamine
- ❏ Pregnyl
- ❏ Procylon
- ❏ Profasi
- ❏ progesterone
- ❏ Repronex
- ❏ Serephene
- ❏ tadalafil
- ❏ Tibolone
- ❏ Uprima
- ❏ urofollitropin
- ❏ Vasomax
- ❏ Viagra
- ❏ Yohimex
- ❏ Yokon

GLAUCOMA

- ❏ acetazolamide
- ❏ AkPro
- ❏ Alphagan
- ❏ Azopt

GLAUCOMA

- ❏ betaxolol
- ❏ Betoptic
- ❏ bimatoprost
- ❏ brimonidine
- ❏ brinzolamide
- ❏ carbachol
- ❏ Carbastat
- ❏ Carboptic
- ❏ Cosopt
- ❏ Daranide
- ❏ demecarium
- ❏ Diamox
- ❏ Diamox Sequels
- ❏ dichlorphenamide
- ❏ dipivefrin
- ❏ dorzolamide
- ❏ echothiophate
- ❏ Epifrin
- ❏ Epinal
- ❏ epinephrine
- ❏ Eppy/N
- ❏ Eserine
- ❏ Floropryl
- ❏ Humorsol
- ❏ isoflurophate
- ❏ isopto carbachol
- ❏ isopto carpine
- ❏ isopto eserine
- ❏ Istalol
- ❏ latanoprost
- ❏ Lumigan
- ❏ Miostat
- ❏ phospholine iodide
- ❏ physostigmine
- ❏ Travatan Z
- ❏ travoprost
- ❏ Trusopt
- ❏ Zalatan

HEMORRHAGE

- ❏ adrenalin chloride
- ❏ Aggrastat
- ❏ albumin
- ❏ AlphaNine SD
- ❏ Amicar
- ❏ aminocaproic acid
- ❏ aprotinin
- ❏ Arixtra
- ❏ Autoplex
- ❏ Avitene
- ❏ BeneFix
- ❏ cellulose, oxidized
- ❏ Corifact
- ❏ Cyklokapron
- ❏ factor IX complex
- ❏ factor XIII
- ❏ Flexbumin
- ❏ gelatin (absorbable)
- ❏ Helistat
- ❏ Hemofil
- ❏ Hemonyne
- ❏ Hemotene
- ❏ Konyne 80
- ❏ Methergine
- ❏ methylergonovine
- ❏ Mononine
- ❏ nimodipine
- ❏ Nimotop
- ❏ NovoSeven
- ❏ Oxycel
- ❏ Profilnine SD
- ❏ Proplex
- ❏ Surgicel
- ❏ thrombin
- ❏ Thrombinar
- ❏ Thrombogen
- ❏ Thrombostat
- ❏ Tirofiban

HEMORRHAGE

- ❏ tranexamic acid
- ❏ Trasylol

MALE DRUGS

- ❏ 5-aminosalicylic acid
- ❏ ABX-EGF
- ❏ alfuzosin
- ❏ alprostadil
- ❏ Andro-Teston
- ❏ Androxal
- ❏ APC8015
- ❏ Asacol
- ❏ Avanafil
- ❏ Aveed
- ❏ Axiron
- ❏ Azo-Gantrisin
- ❏ Avodart
- ❏ Bactrim
- ❏ Baridium
- ❏ biclutamide
- ❏ Buserelin
- ❏ cabazitaxel
- ❏ Canasa
- ❏ Cardura
- ❏ Casodex
- ❏ Caspofungin
- ❏ Caverject
- ❏ Cialis
- ❏ Cotrim
- ❏ Degarelix
- ❏ Delatestryl
- ❏ Depo-Provera
- ❏ Doxazosin
- ❏ dutasteride

MALE DRUGS

- ❏ Eligard
- ❏ Enzyte
- ❏ Exisulind
- ❏ finasteride
- ❏ Flomax
- ❏ Floxin
- ❏ fluoxymesterone
- ❏ Fortesta
- ❏ Fortigel
- ❏ Goserelin
- ❏ Halotestin
- ❏ hydroxythiohomosildenafil
- ❏ Hytrin
- ❏ IFEX
- ❏ Ifosamide
- ❏ Interex
- ❏ Intimex
- ❏ ipilimumab
- ❏ Jalyn
- ❏ Jevtana
- ❏ leuprolide
- ❏ Levitra
- ❏ Livia
- ❏ LoCholest
- ❏ Lupron
- ❏ Maintain
- ❏ ManDelay
- ❏ MasXtreme
- ❏ mesalamine
- ❏ MUSE
- ❏ Nebido
- ❏ Nilandron
- ❏ nilutamide
- ❏ ofloxacin
- ❏ PC SPES
- ❏ PDE5 blocker
- ❏ PDE5 inhibitor

MALE DRUGS

- ❏ Pentasa
- ❏ Phen-Azo
- ❏ phenazopyridine
- ❏ phentolamine
- ❏ phosphodiesterase blocker
- ❏ phosphodiesterase inhibitor
- ❏ phytosterol blocker
- ❏ Prevalite
- ❏ Procylon
- ❏ Prolatis'
- ❏ Proscar
- ❏ prostaglandin E1
- ❏ Provenge
- ❏ pygeum
- ❏ Questran
- ❏ quinolone
- ❏ Revivexxx
- ❏ Rapaflo
- ❏ Rowasa
- ❏ saw palmetto
- ❏ Septra
- ❏ sildenafil citrate
- ❏ silodosin
- ❏ sipuleucel-T
- ❏ Staxyn
- ❏ Striant
- ❏ sulfamethoprim
- ❏ Sulfatrim
- ❏ sulfonamide
- ❏ Suprefact
- ❏ tadalafil
- ❏ tamsulosin
- ❏ terazosin
- ❏ teriparatide
- ❏ testosterone enanthate
- ❏ TimeOut
- ❏ Trelstar
- ❏ Trelstar LA

MALE DRUGS

- ❏ Tribolone
- ❏ triptorelin pamoate
- ❏ Ultra ZN
- ❏ Uprima
- ❏ Urodine
- ❏ Urogesic
- ❏ Uroplus
- ❏ UroXatral
- ❏ Vantas
- ❏ vardenafil
- ❏ VasClip
- ❏ Vasomax
- ❏ Viadur
- ❏ Viagra
- ❏ Vinarol
- ❏ Viridium
- ❏ Yocon
- ❏ Yohimar
- ❏ Yohimbe
- ❏ Yohimbine
- ❏ Zoladex

MUSCLE RELAXANTS

- ❏ abobotulinumtoxinA
- ❏ Amrix
- ❏ Antiflex
- ❏ Ativan
- ❏ Atracurium Besylate
- ❏ baclofen
- ❏ Banflex
- ❏ Blanax
- ❏ Carbacot
- ❏ carisoprodol
- ❏ chlorphenesin
- ❏ chlorzoxazone
- ❏ curare
- ❏ cyclobenzaprine

MUSCLE RELAXANTS

- Dantrium
- Dantrolene
- Delaxin
- diazepam
- Disipal
- Dizac
- Donnatal
- doxacurium chloride
- Dysport
- Flavoxate HCI
- Flaxedil
- Flexagin
- Flexain
- Flexaphen
- Flexeril
- Flexoject
- Flexon
- Gablofen
- gallamine triethiodide
- hexafluorenium
- K-Flex
- Lioresal
- Marbaxin
- Marflex
- mephenesin
- meprobamate
- Mestinon
- metaxalone
- methocarbamol
- metocurine iodide
- Metubine
- Mivacron
- mivacurium chloride
- Myolin
- Myotrol
- Neocyten
- Neostig
- neostigmine

MUSCLE RELAXANTS

- Nimbex
- Noradex
- Norcuron
- Norflex
- Norgesic
- Nuromax
- O-Flex
- Orflagen
- Orfro
- orphenadrine
- orphanagesic
- Orphanate
- Papavirine
- Paraflex
- Parafon
- P-A-V
- phenobarbital
- prostigmin
- pyridostigmine
- Rela
- Relagesic
- Remular
- Robamol
- Robaxin
- Robaxisal
- Robomol
- rocuronium bromide
- Skelaxin
- Skelex
- Sodol
- Soma Compound
- succinylcholine
- Tega-Flex
- tizanidine
- Tracrium
- Tubocurarine
- Urispas
- Valrelease

MUSCLE RELAXANTS

- ❑ vecuronium bromide
- ❑ Zanaflex
- ❑ Zemuron

NEUROLOGY

- ❑ 4-aminopyridine
- ❑ acetazolamide
- ❑ Adderall
- ❑ algalsidase alfa
- ❑ Akineton
- ❑ alglucosidase alfa
- ❑ Alsuma
- ❑ Amantadine
- ❑ Ambenonium
- ❑ Amerge
- ❑ amobarbital
- ❑ amytal
- ❑ Antegren
- ❑ Ampyra
- ❑ Apokyn
- ❑ apomorphine hydrochloride
- ❑ Aricept
- ❑ armodafinil
- ❑ Artane
- ❑ Atamet
- ❑ Atretol
- ❑ Aubagio
- ❑ Avonex
- ❑ Azilect
- ❑ Banzel
- ❑ belimumab
- ❑ Benadryl
- ❑ Benlysta
- ❑ benzetropine mesylate
- ❑ Betaseron
- ❑ Biocadren

NEUROLOGY

- ❑ Biperiden
- ❑ Botox
- ❑ Bromocriptine
- ❑ carbamazepine
- ❑ Carbatrol
- ❑ Carbex
- ❑ carbidopa/levodopa
- ❑ carisbamate
- ❑ Celontin
- ❑ Cerebyx
- ❑ Cevimeline
- ❑ cladribine
- ❑ Clindets
- ❑ clobazam
- ❑ clonazepam
- ❑ clorazepate
- ❑ Cogentin
- ❑ Cognex
- ❑ COMFYDE
- ❑ Concerta
- ❑ Copaxone
- ❑ corticotropin
- ❑ Cuyposa
- ❑ Cylert
- ❑ Cymbalta
- ❑ D-23129
- ❑ dalfampridine
- ❑ Dantrium
- ❑ DaTscan
- ❑ Decadron
- ❑ Deltasone
- ❑ Depacon
- ❑ Depakene
- ❑ Depakote
- ❑ Depo-Medrol
- ❑ Desoxyn
- ❑ dexamethasone
- ❑ Dexedrine

NEUROLOGY

- ❑ Dextrostat
- ❑ dextroamphetamine sulfate
- ❑ DHE 45
- ❑ Diamox
- ❑ difluprednate
- ❑ dihydroergotamine
- ❑ Dilantin
- ❑ diphenhydramine
- ❑ Diphenylan
- ❑ divalproex sodium
- ❑ donepezil
- ❑ Dopram
- ❑ Dornase Alfa
- ❑ duloxetine
- ❑ Durezol
- ❑ Edluar
- ❑ edrophonium chloride
- ❑ Eldepryl
- ❑ Epitol
- ❑ Epsol
- ❑ Ergomar
- ❑ ergotamine
- ❑ eslicarbazepine acetate
- ❑ Estorra
- ❑ eszopiclone
- ❑ ethosuximide
- ❑ Ethotoin
- ❑ Evoxac
- ❑ Exelon
- ❑ Extavia
- ❑ ezogabine
- ❑ Fampridine-SR
- ❑ Felbamate
- ❑ Felbatol
- ❑ fingolimod
- ❑ fosphenytoin
- ❑ FTY720
- ❑ gabapentin

NEUROLOGY

- ❑ gabapentin enacarbil
- ❑ Gabitril
- ❑ Gamunex
- ❑ Gamunex-C
- ❑ Gen-Xene
- ❑ Gilenya
- ❑ glycopyrrolate
- ❑ Gralise
- ❑ Haldol
- ❑ Halperidol
- ❑ HepaGam B
- ❑ Horizant
- ❑ H.P. Acthar Gel
- ❑ hydroxychloroquine
- ❑ Imitrex
- ❑ Increlex
- ❑ Inderal
- ❑ interferon
- ❑ interferon beta-1A
- ❑ interferon beta-1B
- ❑ Intermezzo
- ❑ Invega
- ❑ isoxsuprine
- ❑ JZP-6
- ❑ Kemadrin
- ❑ Keppra
- ❑ Klonopin
- ❑ lacosamide
- ❑ Lamictal
- ❑ Lamictal XR
- ❑ lamotrigine
- ❑ lanreotide acetate
- ❑ Larodopa
- ❑ Levadex
- ❑ Levbid
- ❑ levetiracetam
- ❑ Levsin
- ❑ Levsinex

NEUROLOGY

- ☐ lisdexamfetamine dimesylate
- ☐ Lodosyn
- ☐ loflupane
- ☐ Luminal
- ☐ Lumizyme
- ☐ Lunesta
- ☐ Lyrica
- ☐ magnesium sulfate
- ☐ Maxalt
- ☐ Mebaral
- ☐ mecasermin
- ☐ Medrol
- ☐ Mephenytoin
- ☐ mephobarbital
- ☐ Mesantoin
- ☐ Mestinon
- ☐ methamphetamine
- ☐ Methsuximide
- ☐ methylphenidate
- ☐ methylprednisolone
- ☐ Midrin
- ☐ midocrine
- ☐ Migranal nasal spray
- ☐ milnacipran
- ☐ Milontin
- ☐ Mirapex
- ☐ Mirapex ER
- ☐ Modafinil
- ☐ Myozyme
- ☐ Mysoline
- ☐ Mytelase caplets
- ☐ naratriptan
- ☐ Nascobal
- ☐ natalizumab
- ☐ Neostigmine
- ☐ Neupro
- ☐ Neurontin
- ☐ Novantrone

NEUROLOGY

- ☐ Novo-Clobazam
- ☐ Nuvigil
- ☐ onabotulinumtoxinA
- ☐ Onfi
- ☐ Orap
- ☐ Orapred
- ☐ Orasone
- ☐ oxazepam
- ☐ oxcarbazepine
- ☐ Oxytrol
- ☐ paliperidone
- ☐ Parcopa
- ☐ Parlodel
- ☐ Pediapred
- ☐ Peganone
- ☐ Pemoline
- ☐ Perampanel
- ☐ Pergolide
- ☐ Permax
- ☐ phenobarbital
- ☐ phensuximide
- ☐ Phenytek
- ☐ Phenytoin
- ☐ Pimozide
- ☐ Plaquenil
- ☐ Potiga
- ☐ pramipexole
- ☐ prednisolone
- ☐ prednisone
- ☐ pregabalin
- ☐ Prestara
- ☐ Primidone
- ☐ ProAmatine
- ☐ propranolol
- ☐ Prostigmin
- ☐ Provigil
- ☐ Pulmozyme
- ☐ Pyridostigmine

NEUROLOGY

- ❏ ramelteon
- ❏ rasagiline mesylate
- ❏ Rebif
- ❏ Regonol
- ❏ Replagal
- ❏ Requip
- ❏ Retigabine
- ❏ Rilutek
- ❏ Riluzole
- ❏ rivastigmine
- ❏ rizatriptan
- ❏ ropinirole
- ❏ rotigotine
- ❏ Rozerem
- ❏ rufinamide
- ❏ Sabril
- ❏ Savella
- ❏ Selegiline
- ❏ Sinemet
- ❏ sodium oxybate
- ❏ Solu-Medrol
- ❏ Solzira
- ❏ Somatuline Autogel
- ❏ Somatuline Depot
- ❏ Stalevo
- ❏ Stavzor
- ❏ Stedesa
- ❏ Sublinox
- ❏ succinimide
- ❏ sumatriptan
- ❏ Sumavel DosePro
- ❏ Symmetrel
- ❏ Tacrine
- ❏ Tafamidis
- ❏ Tasmar
- ❏ Tegretol
- ❏ Tensilon

NEUROLOGY

- ❏ Tercica
- ❏ tetrabenazine
- ❏ tiagabine
- ❏ timolol maleate
- ❏ tizanidine
- ❏ TOBI
- ❏ Tobramycin
- ❏ Tolcapone
- ❏ Topamax
- ❏ topiramate
- ❏ Tranxene
- ❏ Tridione
- ❏ trihexyphenidyl
- ❏ Trileptal
- ❏ trimethadione
- ❏ TVP-1012
- ❏ Tysabri
- ❏ Valium
- ❏ valproic acid
- ❏ velaglucerase alfa
- ❏ vigabatrin
- ❏ Vimpat
- ❏ VPRIV
- ❏ Vyvanse
- ❏ Wigraine
- ❏ Xenazine
- ❏ XP13512
- ❏ Xyrem
- ❏ Zanaflex
- ❏ Zarontin
- ❏ Zelapar
- ❏ Zolmitriptan
- ❏ zolpidem
- ❏ Zolpimist
- ❏ Zomig
- ❏ Zonegran
- ❏ zonisamide

OBESITY

- ❏ Acomplia
- ❏ Adipex
- ❏ Adipex-P
- ❏ Adipost
- ❏ Adphen
- ❏ AdvantEdge
- ❏ Alli
- ❏ Anorex
- ❏ Anoxine
- ❏ Appecon
- ❏ Aqua-Ban
- ❏ Axokine
- ❏ AYDS
- ❏ benzphetamine
- ❏ BioLean
- ❏ BioMD Nutraceuticals
- ❏ Biotest Hot-Rox
- ❏ Bontril PDM
- ❏ Carb Cutter
- ❏ Chroma Slim
- ❏ Contrave
- ❏ Dapex
- ❏ desoxyn
- ❏ Dexatrim
- ❏ dexfenfluramine
- ❏ Didrex
- ❏ diethylpropion
- ❏ Dital
- ❏ Dyrexan
- ❏ EAS Thermo DynamX
- ❏ Estrin-D
- ❏ Exgest LA
- ❏ fenfluramine
- ❏ Fen-Phen
- ❏ Hydroxycut
- ❏ Ionamin
- ❏ Isatori Lean
- ❏ Leptoprin

OBESITY

- ❏ LipoTrim
- ❏ Lorcaserin
- ❏ Mazindol
- ❏ Mazinor
- ❏ Medifast
- ❏ Meridia
- ❏ Metab-O-Fx
- ❏ Metabolife
- ❏ methamphetamine
- ❏ MHP TakeOff Hi-Energy
- ❏ M-Orexic
- ❏ Natrol
- ❏ Natrol CitriMax
- ❏ Nature's Bounty Xtreme Lean
- ❏ Nunaturals LevelRight
- ❏ Obalan
- ❏ Obenix
- ❏ Obe-Del
- ❏ Obe-Mar
- ❏ Obe-Nix
- ❏ Obephen
- ❏ Obermine
- ❏ Obestin
- ❏ Obezine
- ❏ Oby-Cap
- ❏ Oby-Trim
- ❏ One-A-Day Weight Smart
- ❏ Orlistat
- ❏ Panrexin
- ❏ Panshape
- ❏ Parzine
- ❏ PatentLean
- ❏ Phendiet
- ❏ phendimetrazine
- ❏ Phentercot
- ❏ phentermine
- ❏ Phentra
- ❏ Phentride

OBESITY

- ❑ Phentrol
- ❑ phenylpropanolamine
- ❑ Phenzine
- ❑ Plegine
- ❑ Pondimin
- ❑ Prelu-2
- ❑ Preludin-Endurete
- ❑ Prolab
- ❑ PT-105
- ❑ PureTrim
- ❑ Qnexa
- ❑ Redux
- ❑ Rexigen
- ❑ rimonabant
- ❑ Sanorex
- ❑ sibutramine
- ❑ Slynn-LL
- ❑ Solo Slim
- ❑ Stacker 2
- ❑ Statobex
- ❑ T-Diet
- ❑ Tega-Nil
- ❑ Tenuate
- ❑ Tenuate Dospan
- ❑ Tepanil
- ❑ Teramin
- ❑ Tetrazene ES-50
- ❑ Thermogenics
- ❑ Thinz
- ❑ ThyroStart
- ❑ Trimstat
- ❑ Twinlab GTB Chromium
- ❑ Wehles
- ❑ Wehles Timecelles
- ❑ Weightrol
- ❑ Xenadrine
- ❑ Xenical
- ❑ XtremeLean

OBESITY

- ❑ X-Trozine LA
- ❑ Zantrex
- ❑ Zantryl

OB/GYN

- ❑ 17-beta estradiol
- ❑ acid jelly
- ❑ Aci-Jel
- ❑ Aclasta
- ❑ Activella
- ❑ Activelle
- ❑ Actonel
- ❑ acyclovir
- ❑ adalimumab
- ❑ Adipex
- ❑ Adipex-P
- ❑ Adriana
- ❑ Aldara
- ❑ alendronate
- ❑ Alesse
- ❑ Alluna
- ❑ Alora
- ❑ Amen
- ❑ Amerge
- ❑ amphotericin
- ❑ anastrozole
- ❑ Ancobon
- ❑ Angeliq
- ❑ anidulafungin
- ❑ A.P.L.
- ❑ Apri
- ❑ ArginMax
- ❑ Arimidex
- ❑ Atelvia
- ❑ AVC Cream
- ❑ Aviane

OB/GYN

- ❏ Avlimil
- ❏ Aygestin
- ❏ Azactim
- ❏ AZO
- ❏ Bactrim
- ❏ Betadine
- ❏ Beyaz
- ❏ Bijuva
- ❏ Bio-E-Gel
- ❏ Boniva
- ❏ Brevicon
- ❏ bromocriptine
- ❏ BufferGel
- ❏ butoconazole
- ❏ Cacit
- ❏ calcitonin
- ❏ Calcitonin-Salmon
- ❏ Cancidas
- ❏ Canesten
- ❏ carboprost
- ❏ Carlesta
- ❏ caspofungin
- ❏ Cellasene
- ❏ Cenestin
- ❏ Ceptaz
- ❏ Cervidil
- ❏ Cetrorelix
- ❏ Cetrotide
- ❏ cholecalciferol
- ❏ chorionic gonadotropin
- ❏ Cipro
- ❏ ciprofloxacin
- ❏ CitraNatal
- ❏ Clearblue
- ❏ Cleocin
- ❏ Climara
- ❏ Climara Pro
- ❏ Clindesse

OB/GYN

- ❏ Clomid
- ❏ clomiphene citrate
- ❏ Clotrimaderm
- ❏ clotrimazole
- ❏ CombiPatch
- ❏ Conceptrol
- ❏ Condylox
- ❏ Crinone
- ❏ Cyclen
- ❏ Cyclessa
- ❏ Cycrin
- ❏ Cryselle
- ❏ Cystex
- ❏ Cystospas
- ❏ DawnMist
- ❏ DDAVP
- ❏ Delestrogen
- ❏ Delfen
- ❏ Demulin
- ❏ denosumab
- ❏ Depo-Provera
- ❏ depo-sub✈ provera
- ❏ Desmopressin
- ❏ Desogen
- ❏ desogestrel
- ❏ desvenlafaxine
- ❏ Detrol
- ❏ Detrol LA
- ❏ D.H.E.
- ❏ dienestrol
- ❏ Diflucan
- ❏ dihydroergotamine
- ❏ dinoprostone
- ❏ Divigel
- ❏ dong quai
- ❏ drospirenone
- ❏ Duralutin
- ❏ Duricef

OB/GYN

- ❏ EC-Naprosyn
- ❏ econazole
- ❏ Ecostatin
- ❏ Edex
- ❏ eflornithine
- ❏ Elestrin
- ❏ Ellence
- ❏ EMKO
- ❏ Enjuvia
- ❏ Enovid
- ❏ Enpresse
- ❏ Epirubicin
- ❏ Eraxis
- ❏ Ergomar
- ❏ ergotamine tartrate
- ❏ Esclim Patch
- ❏ Essure
- ❏ Estinyl
- ❏ Estrace
- ❏ Estraderm
- ❏ estradiol
- ❏ Estrasorb
- ❏ Estratab
- ❏ Estratest
- ❏ Estratest H.S.
- ❏ Estring
- ❏ EstroGel
- ❏ estrogen
- ❏ estropipate
- ❏ Estrostep
- ❏ ethyl estradiol
- ❏ ethynodiol diacetate
- ❏ Euthoid
- ❏ Evamist
- ❏ Evista
- ❏ Extrasorb
- ❏ Fablyn
- ❏ famciclovir

OB/GYN

- ❏ Famvir
- ❏ Fareston
- ❏ Faslodex
- ❏ FDS feminine spray
- ❏ Femara
- ❏ Fem-Cap
- ❏ FemCare
- ❏ Femcet
- ❏ Femhrt
- ❏ Femizol
- ❏ Fempatch
- ❏ Femring
- ❏ Femstat
- ❏ Femtrace
- ❏ Fertinex
- ❏ Flibanserin
- ❏ flucytosine
- ❏ fluoxetine
- ❏ Follistim
- ❏ follitropin alfa/beta
- ❏ Fortaz
- ❏ Forteo
- ❏ Fortical
- ❏ Fosamax
- ❏ Fosteum
- ❏ fulvestrant
- ❏ Fungizone
- ❏ Furadantin
- ❏ Gardasil
- ❏ Genapax
- ❏ GenCept
- ❏ genistein aglycone
- ❏ Genora
- ❏ gentian violet
- ❏ Gesterol
- ❏ Gestiva
- ❏ Gonal
- ❏ Gynazole

OB/GYN

- GyneCure
- Gyne-Lotrimin
- Gynix
- Gynodiol
- Gyno-Trosyd
- Hemabate
- Herceptin
- Humegon
- Humira
- hydroxyprogesterone caproate
- Hy/Gestrone
- Hylutin
- HypRho
- Hyprogest
- Hyproval P.A.
- Hyskon
- ibandronate
- imiquimod
- Imitrex
- incobotulinumtoxinA
- Indocin
- indomethacin
- Innofem
- Inti-Mist
- Intrinsa
- itraconazole
- ixabepilone
- Ixempra
- Jadelle
- Jenest
- Junel
- Kariva
- ketoconazole
- Koo Sar
- Koromex
- lanreotide acetate
- lapatinib
- lasofoxifene

OB/GYN

- Legatrin PM
- Lessina
- letrozole
- Levaquin
- Levlen
- Levlite
- levomefolate
- levonorgestrel
- Levora
- Levothroid
- levothyroxine
- Levoxyl
- LibiGel
- Liotrix
- Lippes Loop
- Liquibeads
- Loestrin
- Lo/Ovral
- Low-Ogestrel
- Lubriderm
- Lunelle
- Lupron
- Lutera
- lutropin alfa
- Luveris
- Lybrel
- Lysteda
- Macrobid
- Macrodantin
- Makena
- Marvelon
- Massengil products
- Maxalt
- Maxipime
- medroxyprogesterone
- Megace
- Menest
- Menocheck

OB/GYN

- ❏ Menostar
- ❏ mentropin
- ❏ Mestranol
- ❏ metazoline
- ❏ Methergine
- ❏ Metrodin
- ❏ MetroGel
- ❏ metronidazole
- ❏ Miacalcin
- ❏ miconazole
- ❏ MICRhoGAM
- ❏ Micronor
- ❏ Midol
- ❏ Mifeprex
- ❏ mifepristone
- ❏ MigraHealth
- ❏ Migranal
- ❏ Minestrin
- ❏ Minoxidil
- ❏ Min-Ovral
- ❏ Mircette
- ❏ Mirena
- ❏ ModiCon
- ❏ Monistat
- ❏ Monistat 3
- ❏ Monistat 7
- ❏ Mono-Stat
- ❏ Monuril
- ❏ MUSE
- ❏ Mycelex
- ❏ Myclo
- ❏ Myclo-Gyne
- ❏ Mycostatin
- ❏ M-Zole 3
- ❏ Nadostine
- ❏ Nafarelin
- ❏ naladixic acid
- ❏ naratriptan

OB/GYN

- ❏ Necon
- ❏ N.E.E.
- ❏ NegGram
- ❏ Nelova
- ❏ Nelulen
- ❏ Neutrogena products
- ❏ Nicomide
- ❏ Nicosyn
- ❏ nicotinamide
- ❏ Nilstat
- ❏ Nizoral A-D
- ❏ Nolvadex
- ❏ nonoxynol-9
- ❏ Norcept
- ❏ Nordette
- ❏ norelgestromin
- ❏ norethindrone
- ❏ Norforms
- ❏ Norgestrel
- ❏ Norinyl
- ❏ Norlutate
- ❏ Norlutin
- ❏ Noroxin
- ❏ Norplant
- ❏ Nor-QD
- ❏ Nortrel
- ❏ Novo-Miconazole
- ❏ Noxafil
- ❏ NuvaRing
- ❏ Nyaderm
- ❏ Nystatin
- ❏ Ogen cream
- ❏ Ogestrel
- ❏ Ortho-Cept
- ❏ Ortho-Creme
- ❏ Ortho-Cyclen
- ❏ Ortho Dienestrol
- ❏ Ortho-Est

OB/GYN

- ❏ Ortho Evra Patch
- ❏ Ortho-Gynol
- ❏ Ortho-Micronor
- ❏ Ortho-Novum
- ❏ Ortho-Prefest
- ❏ Ortho Tri-Cyclen
- ❏ Ortho Tri-Cyclen Lo
- ❏ Osteo Bi-Flex
- ❏ OvaRex
- ❏ Ovcon
- ❏ Ovidrel
- ❏ Ovral
- ❏ Ovrette
- ❏ oxytocin
- ❏ Oxytrol
- ❏ Pamprin
- ❏ papillomavirus
- ❏ ParaGard T380a
- ❏ Parlodel
- ❏ Pediapred
- ❏ Pediarix
- ❏ Penlac polish
- ❏ Pennsaid
- ❏ Pergonal
- ❏ phytoestrogen
- ❏ piperazine estrone
- ❏ Pitocin
- ❏ Pitressin
- ❏ Plan B
- ❏ Plan B One-Step
- ❏ podofilux gel
- ❏ Portia
- ❏ posaconazole
- ❏ prednisolone
- ❏ prednisone
- ❏ Pregnyl
- ❏ Premarin
- ❏ Premphase

OB/GYN

- ❏ Prempro
- ❏ Premsyn
- ❏ Prepidil
- ❏ Prestara
- ❏ Primaxin
- ❏ Pristiq
- ❏ Prochieve
- ❏ Pro-Depo
- ❏ Progestaject
- ❏ progesterone
- ❏ progesterone gel
- ❏ Progestilin
- ❏ Prolia
- ❏ Proloid
- ❏ Prometrium
- ❏ Prosed
- ❏ prostaglandine
- ❏ Prostin E2
- ❏ Provera
- ❏ Psorcon
- ❏ Pyridium
- ❏ quadrivalent
- ❏ Radiance injection
- ❏ Raloxifene
- ❏ Reclast
- ❏ RepHresh
- ❏ Replens
- ❏ Repronex
- ❏ RespiGam
- ❏ risedronate
- ❏ ritodrine
- ❏ rizatriptan
- ❏ Rovamycine
- ❏ RU-486
- ❏ Sarafem
- ❏ SCE-A
- ❏ Sedapap
- ❏ Semicid

OB/GYN

- ❏ Septra
- ❏ Soltamox
- ❏ Somatuline
- ❏ Spiramycin
- ❏ Sporanox
- ❏ Sultran
- ❏ sumatriptan
- ❏ Sumavel DosePro
- ❏ Summer's Eve
- ❏ Symphasic
- ❏ Synarel
- ❏ Synthroid
- ❏ Syntocinon
- ❏ tamoxifen
- ❏ Terazol
- ❏ teriparatide
- ❏ testolactone
- ❏ ThermaCare
- ❏ ThinPrep
- ❏ Tindamax
- ❏ tinidazole
- ❏ tioconazole
- ❏ Tolterodine
- ❏ toremifene
- ❏ tranexamic acid
- ❏ Tri-Levlen
- ❏ Tri-Norinyl
- ❏ Triphasil
- ❏ Tri-Sprintec
- ❏ Trivora
- ❏ Tropsium
- ❏ Tykerb
- ❏ Urised
- ❏ Urobiotic
- ❏ urofollitropin
- ❏ Uroquid
- ❏ Vagifem
- ❏ Vagisil

OB/GYN

- ❏ Vagistat
- ❏ valacyclovir
- ❏ Valtrex
- ❏ Vaniqa
- ❏ Vasopressin
- ❏ Venastat
- ❏ Viactiv
- ❏ Viagra
- ❏ Vivelle-Dot
- ❏ Wigraine
- ❏ WinRho SDF
- ❏ Xeomin
- ❏ Yokon
- ❏ Yutopar
- ❏ Zaroxolyn
- ❏ zoledronic acid
- ❏ zolmitriptan
- ❏ Zomig
- ❏ Zovia
- ❏ Zovirax

OPHTHALMICS

- ❏ acetazolamide
- ❏ acetylcholine
- ❏ Acular
- ❏ Acuvail
- ❏ Adsorbocarpine
- ❏ aflibercept
- ❏ Akarpine
- ❏ AK-Con
- ❏ AK-Dilate
- ❏ AK-Fluor
- ❏ AK-Nefrin
- ❏ AK-Pentolate
- ❏ AK-Poly-Bac
- ❏ AK-Pred

OPHTHALMICS

- AK-Spore
- Akten
- Aktob
- AK-Tracin
- AK-Trol
- Akwa Tears
- Alaway
- alcaftadine
- Alcaine
- Almocarpine
- Alomide
- alpha chymar
- alpha chymotrypsin
- alpha lipoic
- Alrex
- Anacel
- Antibiopto
- Aosoft
- apraclonidine
- Aquify
- Atropine
- AzaSite
- azithromycin
- Azopt
- bacitracin
- Benoxinate
- benzalkonium
- bepotastine
- Bepreve
- besifloxacin
- Besivance
- Betaxon
- Betoptic
- bimatoprost
- Bion Tears
- Bleph-10
- Blephamide
- Blink

OPHTHALMICS

- Blinx
- Botox
- brimonidine tartrate
- brinzolamide
- Bromday
- bromfenac
- BSS
- Bufopto
- Carbacel
- Carbachol
- Caterase
- Cetapred
- Chibroxin
- chloramphenicol
- Chloromycetin
- Chloroptic
- chymotrypsin
- Ciloxan
- Clear Care
- Clear Eyes
- Clerz
- Collyrium
- Coly-Mycin
- Combigan
- Complete
- Cortisporin
- cromolyn sodium
- Cromoptic
- Cyclogyl
- cyclopentolate
- cycloplegic
- Cysteamine
- Dacriose
- dapiprazole
- Daranide
- Definity
- Degest
- demacarium

OPHTHALMICS

- ❑ dexamethasone
- ❑ Diamox
- ❑ dichlorphenamide
- ❑ difluprednate
- ❑ Dilatair
- ❑ Dionephrine
- ❑ diquafosol tetrasodium
- ❑ Dorsolamide
- ❑ DuoVisc
- ❑ Duratears
- ❑ Durezol
- ❑ E-Carpine
- ❑ Ecodide
- ❑ Econochlor
- ❑ Econopred
- ❑ Efricel
- ❑ Elestat
- ❑ Emedastine
- ❑ Emidine
- ❑ Enuclene
- ❑ E-Pilo
- ❑ Epinal
- ❑ epinastine hydrochloride
- ❑ erythromycin ethylsuccinate
- ❑ ethoxzolamide
- ❑ Eyesine
- ❑ Eylea
- ❑ Fluoracaine
- ❑ fluorescein
- ❑ fluorometholone
- ❑ Fluoroseptic
- ❑ Fluress
- ❑ FML
- ❑ Fomivirsen
- ❑ Ful-Glo
- ❑ Funduscein
- ❑ ganciclovir
- ❑ gatifloxacin

OPHTHALMICS

- ❑ Gentak
- ❑ gentamicin
- ❑ GenTeal
- ❑ Glaucon
- ❑ glutathione
- ❑ Herplex
- ❑ HMS Liquifilm
- ❑ Homatrocel
- ❑ Humorsol
- ❑ hyaluronidase
- ❑ hydroxypropyl
- ❑ Hy-Flo
- ❑ Hylenex
- ❑ Hypersal
- ❑ hypromellose
- ❑ IC-Green
- ❑ Iluvien
- ❑ idoxuridine
- ❑ Ilotycin
- ❑ indocyanine green
- ❑ Inflamase
- ❑ INS365
- ❑ IntraLase
- ❑ Iopidine
- ❑ I-Phrine
- ❑ Iquix
- ❑ Irigate
- ❑ Isopto atropine
- ❑ Isopto carbachol
- ❑ Isopto cetamide
- ❑ Isopto eserine
- ❑ Istalol
- ❑ ketorolac tromethamine
- ❑ ketotifen
- ❑ Lacri-Lube
- ❑ Lacrisert
- ❑ Lasik eye surgery
- ❑ Lastacaft

OPHTHALMICS

- ❑ Latisse
- ❑ levobetaxolol
- ❑ levobunolol
- ❑ levofloxacin
- ❑ Lopidine
- ❑ Lotemax
- ❑ Loteprednol
- ❑ lodoxamide
- ❑ Lucentis
- ❑ Lumigan
- ❑ Luveniq
- ❑ LX211
- ❑ Lytears
- ❑ Macugen
- ❑ Medimyd
- ❑ medrysone
- ❑ Methopto
- ❑ Methulose
- ❑ methylcellulose
- ❑ Metreton
- ❑ Miocarpine
- ❑ Miochol
- ❑ Mi-Pilo
- ❑ Murine
- ❑ Muro 128
- ❑ Muro Gonio-Gel
- ❑ Muro ointment
- ❑ Murocoll
- ❑ Mydriacyl
- ❑ Mydrin
- ❑ Mytrate
- ❑ naphazoline
- ❑ Naphcon A
- ❑ Navstel
- ❑ NeoDecadron
- ❑ Neo-Flo
- ❑ Neo-Frin
- ❑ Neomycin

OPHTHALMICS

- ❑ Neo-Synephrine
- ❑ Neozin
- ❑ nepafenac
- ❑ Nevanac
- ❑ Ocu-Carpine
- ❑ Ocu-Mycin
- ❑ Ocu-Phrin
- ❑ Ocuflox
- ❑ OcuFresh
- ❑ Ocugestrin
- ❑ OcuGuard
- ❑ OcuHist
- ❑ Ocusert Pilo
- ❑ OCuSOFT
- ❑ Ocusol
- ❑ olopatadine
- ❑ onabotulinumtoxinA
- ❑ Opcon-A
- ❑ Ophthaine
- ❑ Ophthetic
- ❑ Ophthochlor
- ❑ Ophthocort
- ❑ Opticrom
- ❑ Opti-Free
- ❑ OptiGold
- ❑ Optimyd
- ❑ Optipranolol
- ❑ Optised
- ❑ Optivar
- ❑ Optive
- ❑ Ozurdex
- ❑ papain
- ❑ Pataday
- ❑ Patanol
- ❑ pegaptanib
- ❑ Pemirolast
- ❑ Pereflutren Lipid
- ❑ pheniramine maleate

OPHTHALMICS

- ❏ Phenoptic
- ❏ phenylephrine
- ❏ Phospholine
- ❏ Pilocar
- ❏ Pilocarpine
- ❏ Pilocel
- ❏ Pilopine
- ❏ Piloptic
- ❏ Pilostat
- ❏ Polytrim
- ❏ prednisolone
- ❏ prednisone
- ❏ Predulose
- ❏ Prefrin
- ❏ Proparacaine
- ❏ propylene glycol
- ❏ P.V. Carpine
- ❏ Quixin
- ❏ ranibizumab
- ❏ Refresh Celluvisc
- ❏ Refresh Liquigel
- ❏ Refresh Optive
- ❏ Refresh P.M.
- ❏ Refresh Tears
- ❏ ReNu
- ❏ Restasis
- ❏ Retisert
- ❏ Rev-Eyes
- ❏ Rohto Hydra
- ❏ Rohto V
- ❏ Rohto Zi
- ❏ Rose Bengal
- ❏ Saflutan
- ❏ Salagen
- ❏ silver nitrate
- ❏ Soothe XP
- ❏ Spersaphrine
- ❏ SteriLid

OPHTHALMICS

- ❏ Stoxil
- ❏ Stye
- ❏ Sulfacel
- ❏ sulfacetamide
- ❏ Systane
- ❏ tafluprost
- ❏ Tearisol
- ❏ Tears Naturale
- ❏ Tetracaine
- ❏ tetracycline
- ❏ tetrahydrozoline
- ❏ TheraTears
- ❏ timolol
- ❏ Timoptic
- ❏ Timoptic-XE
- ❏ Travatan Z
- ❏ travoprost
- ❏ triamcinolone
- ❏ tricarbocyanine
- ❏ Triesence
- ❏ trifluorothymidine
- ❏ Trivaris
- ❏ tropicamide
- ❏ Trusopt
- ❏ tyloxapol
- ❏ Ultrazyme
- ❏ Unisol 4
- ❏ Vasocidin
- ❏ Vasocon
- ❏ Vasosulf
- ❏ verteporfin
- ❏ vidarabine
- ❏ Vira-A
- ❏ Virasert
- ❏ Viroptic
- ❏ Visine
- ❏ Visine-A
- ❏ Visine A.C.

OPHTHALMICS

- ❏ Visine L.R.
- ❏ Visine Tears
- ❏ Visculose
- ❏ Visudyne
- ❏ VISUtein
- ❏ VISX
- ❏ Vitravene
- ❏ Viva-Drops
- ❏ wavefront-guided laser
- ❏ Xibrom
- ❏ XiDay
- ❏ Zaditor
- ❏ zeaxanthin
- ❏ zinc bacitracin
- ❏ Zincfren
- ❏ zinc sulfate
- ❏ Zirgan
- ❏ Zolyse
- ❏ Zylet
- ❏ Zymaxid

PARKINSON'S

- ❏ Akineton
- ❏ amantadine hydrochloride
- ❏ Apokyn
- ❏ apomorphine hydrochloride
- ❏ Azilect
- ❏ Benadryl
- ❏ benztropine
- ❏ biperiden hydrochloride
- ❏ bromocriptine mesylate
- ❏ cabergoline
- ❏ carbidopa
- ❏ carbidopa-levodopa
- ❏ Cogentin

PARKINSON'S

- ❏ Comtan
- ❏ DaTscan
- ❏ diphenhydramine hydrochloride
- ❏ Dostinex
- ❏ droxidopa
- ❏ Eldepryl
- ❏ entacapone
- ❏ gabapentin
- ❏ ioflupane
- ❏ Kemadrin
- ❏ levodopa
- ❏ Lodosyn
- ❏ memantine hydrochloride
- ❏ Mirapex
- ❏ Mirapex ER
- ❏ Namenda
- ❏ Neurontin
- ❏ Norflex
- ❏ Northera
- ❏ orphenadrine
- ❏ Parcopa
- ❏ Parlodel
- ❏ pergolide
- ❏ Permax
- ❏ pramipexole dihydrochloride
- ❏ procyclidine hydrochloride
- ❏ rasagiline
- ❏ Requip
- ❏ ropinirole hydrochloride
- ❏ selegiline hydrochloride
- ❏ Sinemet
- ❏ Sinemet CR
- ❏ Stalevo
- ❏ Symmetrel
- ❏ Tasmar
- ❏ tolcapone
- ❏ trihexyphenidyl

PSYCHOTROPICS

- ❑ Abilify
- ❑ Abilify Discmelt
- ❑ Adasuve
- ❑ alprazolam
- ❑ Ambien
- ❑ amitriptyline
- ❑ amoxapine
- ❑ amphetamine
- ❑ Anafranil
- ❑ Aplenzin
- ❑ aripiprazole
- ❑ asenapine
- ❑ Asendin
- ❑ Atarax
- ❑ Ativan
- ❑ atomoxetine
- ❑ AZ-004
- ❑ barbiturate
- ❑ Benzedrine
- ❑ benzodiazepine
- ❑ bromazepam
- ❑ bupropion
- ❑ Buspar
- ❑ buspirone
- ❑ butabarbital
- ❑ Butisol
- ❑ carbamazepine
- ❑ Campral
- ❑ Celexa
- ❑ Centrax
- ❑ Chantix
- ❑ chloral hydrate
- ❑ chlordiazepoxide
- ❑ chlorpromazine
- ❑ Ciltyri
- ❑ Citalopram
- ❑ Clindex
- ❑ Clinoxide

PSYCHOTROPICS

- ❑ clomipramine
- ❑ clonazepam
- ❑ Clonicel
- ❑ clorazepate
- ❑ clozapine
- ❑ Clozaril
- ❑ Compazine
- ❑ Concerta
- ❑ Connexyn
- ❑ Cylert
- ❑ Cymbalta
- ❑ Dalmane
- ❑ Daytrana
- ❑ Depakote
- ❑ desipramine
- ❑ Desoxyn
- ❑ desvenlafaxine
- ❑ Desyrel
- ❑ Dexedrine
- ❑ dexmethylphenidate
- ❑ Diastat
- ❑ diazepam
- ❑ Doral
- ❑ doxepin
- ❑ Droperidol
- ❑ duloxetine
- ❑ Edluar
- ❑ Effexor
- ❑ Elavil
- ❑ Emsam
- ❑ Endep
- ❑ eplivanserin
- ❑ Equetro
- ❑ escitalopram oxalate
- ❑ Eskalith
- ❑ estazolam
- ❑ Estorra
- ❑ ethchlorvynol

PSYCHOTROPICS

- ❑ Etrafon
- ❑ Fanapt
- ❑ FazaClo
- ❑ flunitrazepam
- ❑ fluoxetine
- ❑ fluvoxamine
- ❑ Focalin XR
- ❑ Geodon
- ❑ guanfacine
- ❑ halazepam
- ❑ Halcion
- ❑ Haldol
- ❑ haloperidol
- ❑ hydrochlorothiazide
- ❑ hydroxyzine pamoate
- ❑ iloperidone
- ❑ imipramine
- ❑ Indiplon
- ❑ Intuniv
- ❑ Invega
- ❑ ketazolam
- ❑ Klonopin
- ❑ Latuda
- ❑ Lexapro
- ❑ Librax
- ❑ Libritabs
- ❑ Librium
- ❑ Lidoxide
- ❑ Limbitrol
- ❑ lisdexamfetamine dimesylate
- ❑ Lithium
- ❑ Lithobid
- ❑ Lopoxide
- ❑ lorazepam
- ❑ loxapine
- ❑ Loxitane
- ❑ LSD
- ❑ Ludiomil

PSYCHOTROPICS

- ❑ Lunesta
- ❑ lurasidone
- ❑ Luvox
- ❑ maprotiline
- ❑ Mebaral
- ❑ Medillium
- ❑ Megace
- ❑ megestrol
- ❑ Mellaril
- ❑ mephobarbital
- ❑ meprobamate
- ❑ mesoridazine
- ❑ methylphenidate
- ❑ Meval
- ❑ midazolam
- ❑ Miltown
- ❑ mirtazapine
- ❑ Moban
- ❑ modafinil
- ❑ molindone
- ❑ MTS
- ❑ nafazodone
- ❑ Nardil
- ❑ Navane
- ❑ Nembutal
- ❑ Nipolept
- ❑ Niravam
- ❑ nitrazepam
- ❑ Norpramin
- ❑ nortriptyline
- ❑ Nu-Alpraz
- ❑ Nu-Loraz
- ❑ olanzapine
- ❑ Oleptro
- ❑ Orap
- ❑ Oretic
- ❑ oxazepam
- ❑ paliperidone

PSYCHOTROPICS

- ❑ Pamelor
- ❑ Parnate
- ❑ paroxetine
- ❑ Paxil
- ❑ Paxil CR
- ❑ Paxipam
- ❑ pentobarbital
- ❑ perphenazine
- ❑ phencyclidine
- ❑ phenelzine
- ❑ phenothiazide
- ❑ Placidyl
- ❑ PMB 200
- ❑ PMS
- ❑ prazepam
- ❑ Pristiq
- ❑ prochlorperazine
- ❑ Prolixin
- ❑ ProSom
- ❑ protriptyline
- ❑ provigil
- ❑ Prozac
- ❑ Quaalude
- ❑ quazepam
- ❑ quetiapine
- ❑ ramelteon
- ❑ Remeron
- ❑ REMERONSolTab
- ❑ Restoril
- ❑ Risperdal
- ❑ Risperdal Consta
- ❑ risperidone
- ❑ Ritalin
- ❑ Rivotril
- ❑ Rohypnol
- ❑ roofie
- ❑ Rozerem
- ❑ Saphris

PSYCHOTROPICS

- ❑ Sarafem
- ❑ Seconal
- ❑ selegiline
- ❑ Sepracor
- ❑ Serax
- ❑ Serdolect
- ❑ Serentil
- ❑ Seroquel
- ❑ Seroquel XR
- ❑ sertindole
- ❑ sertraline
- ❑ Serzone
- ❑ Silenor
- ❑ Sinequan
- ❑ sodium brevital
- ❑ sodium pentothal
- ❑ sodium seconal
- ❑ Solium
- ❑ Somnol
- ❑ Sonata
- ❑ Staccato
- ❑ Stavzor
- ❑ Stelazine
- ❑ Strattera
- ❑ Sublinox
- ❑ Surmontil
- ❑ Symbyax
- ❑ temazepam
- ❑ thiordazine
- ❑ thiothixine
- ❑ Thorazine
- ❑ Tofranil
- ❑ T-Quil
- ❑ Trancopal
- ❑ Tranxene
- ❑ tranylcypromine sulfate
- ❑ trazodone
- ❑ Triavil

PSYCHOTROPICS

- ❑ triazolam
- ❑ Trilafon
- ❑ trimipramine maleate
- ❑ Valium
- ❑ valproic
- ❑ Valrelease
- ❑ varenicline
- ❑ venlafaxine
- ❑ Viibryd
- ❑ vilazodone
- ❑ Vistaril
- ❑ Vivactil
- ❑ Vivol
- ❑ Vyvanse
- ❑ Wellbutrin
- ❑ Xanax
- ❑ Zaleplon
- ❑ Zapex
- ❑ Zenvia
- ❑ Zetran
- ❑ ziprasidone
- ❑ Zoloft
- ❑ zolpidem
- ❑ Zolpimist
- ❑ zotepine
- ❑ Zyprexa
- ❑ Zyprexa Relprevv

SHOCK

- ❑ albumin
- ❑ aminocaproic acid
- ❑ Dalalone
- ❑ Decadron
- ❑ Decaject
- ❑ dexamethasone
- ❑ Dexasone

SHOCK

- ❑ Dexone
- ❑ Dextran
- ❑ dextrose in NaCl
- ❑ dextrose in water
- ❑ dopamine
- ❑ Flexbumin
- ❑ Gentran
- ❑ Hexadrol
- ❑ hydrocortisone
- ❑ Intropin
- ❑ isoproterenol
- ❑ Macrodex
- ❑ methylprednisolone
- ❑ Neo-Synephrine
- ❑ phenylephrine
- ❑ Plasmanate
- ❑ Plasma-Plex
- ❑ plasma protein fraction
- ❑ Plasmatein
- ❑ Protenate
- ❑ Rheomacrodex
- ❑ Solurex

UROLOGY

- ❑ Aci-Jel
- ❑ Aldara
- ❑ aldesleukin
- ❑ allopurinol
- ❑ amino acid injection
- ❑ Aminosyn
- ❑ Amoxil
- ❑ Amphotec
- ❑ amphotericin
- ❑ ampicillin
- ❑ Ancobon
- ❑ Androderm

UROLOGY

- Android
- Andro-L.A.
- Andropository
- Anturol
- Atrosept
- Augmentin
- Azactam
- aztreonam
- Bactrim
- bethanechol
- Bethaprim
- BranchAmin
- bumetanide
- Calcibind
- Capen
- Captimer
- Cardura
- Ceclor
- cefepime
- cefixime
- cefmetazole
- Cefobid
- cefonicid
- cefoperazone
- Ceftin
- ceftizoxime
- cefuroxime
- Ceptaz
- cholesteryl
- Cinobac
- cinoxacin
- Cipro
- ciprofloxacin
- Claforan
- clavulanate
- Clorpactin
- clotrimazole
- Condylox

UROLOGY

- conivaptan
- Cotrim
- Cuprimine
- Cymbalta
- Cystagon
- cysteamine
- Cystospaz
- darifenacin
- DDAVP
- Delatest
- Delatestryl
- depAndro
- Depen
- Depotest
- Depo Testosterone
- desmopressin
- Detrol
- Detrol LA
- dimethyl sulfoxide
- Ditropan
- Ditropan XL
- Dolsed
- Doribax
- doripenem
- Doryx
- doxercalciferol
- duloxetine
- Duratest
- Durathate
- Duricef
- Duvoid
- Elmiron
- Enablex
- Epatiol
- Ethyol
- Everone
- febuxostat
- fesoterodine fumarate

UROLOGY

- ❑ Flomax
- ❑ Flovoxate
- ❑ Fortaz
- ❑ fosfomycin
- ❑ Fosrenol
- ❑ FreAmine
- ❑ Fungizone
- ❑ Furadantin
- ❑ Furalan
- ❑ Furan
- ❑ Furanite
- ❑ gatifloxacin
- ❑ Gelnique
- ❑ Hectorol
- ❑ HepatAmine
- ❑ Hipex
- ❑ Histerone
- ❑ hyaluronidase
- ❑ Hylenex
- ❑ hyoscyamine
- ❑ Hytrin
- ❑ imipenem
- ❑ imiquimod
- ❑ Keflex
- ❑ ketoconazole
- ❑ K-Phos
- ❑ lanthanum carbonate
- ❑ Lithostat
- ❑ leuprolide
- ❑ Levaquin
- ❑ levofloxacin
- ❑ Lorabid
- ❑ Loracarbef
- ❑ Lotrim
- ❑ Lupron
- ❑ Lyphocin
- ❑ Macrobid
- ❑ Macrodantin

UROLOGY

- ❑ Mandelamine
- ❑ Mannitol
- ❑ Maxipime
- ❑ Mesna
- ❑ MESNIX
- ❑ methenamine
- ❑ methyltestosterone
- ❑ mezlocillin
- ❑ Mirabegron
- ❑ Monodox
- ❑ Monurol
- ❑ Mucolysin
- ❑ Mycelex
- ❑ nalidixic acid
- ❑ NegGram
- ❑ Neomycin
- ❑ Neosporin
- ❑ NephrAmine
- ❑ nitrofurantoin
- ❑ Nizoral A-D
- ❑ norfloxacin
- ❑ Noroxin
- ❑ Novamine
- ❑ NuLev
- ❑ ofloxacin
- ❑ Oreton Methyl
- ❑ OTG
- ❑ oxybutynin
- ❑ oxybutynin hydrochloride
- ❑ oxytetracycline
- ❑ penicillamine
- ❑ pentosan polysulfate
- ❑ piperacillin
- ❑ Podocon
- ❑ podofilox
- ❑ Polycitra
- ❑ potassium citrate
- ❑ Primaxin

UROLOGY

- ❏ Primsol
- ❏ ProcalAmine
- ❏ Prodium
- ❏ Proloprim
- ❏ Proquin XR
- ❏ Proscar
- ❏ Prosed
- ❏ Protrin
- ❏ Pyridium
- ❏ Renacidin irrigation
- ❏ Renagel
- ❏ RenAmin
- ❏ Rimso
- ❏ Rocephin
- ❏ Sanctura
- ❏ Sanctura XR
- ❏ Sensipar
- ❏ Septra
- ❏ solifenacin succinate
- ❏ sulfamethoprim
- ❏ Sulfaprim
- ❏ sulfathiazole
- ❏ Sulfoxaprim
- ❏ Sultrin
- ❏ Sutilan
- ❏ Tequin
- ❏ Terazol
- ❏ terconazole
- ❏ Tesamone
- ❏ Testoderm
- ❏ Testopel Pellet
- ❏ Thiola
- ❏ ticarcillin
- ❏ Timentin
- ❏ Tioglis
- ❏ tiopronin
- ❏ tolterodine
- ❏ torsemide

UROLOGY

- ❏ Toviaz
- ❏ Travasol
- ❏ trimethoprim
- ❏ Trimpex
- ❏ TrophAmine
- ❏ trospium
- ❏ trospium chloride
- ❏ Uloric
- ❏ Urecholine
- ❏ Urex
- ❏ Uricalm
- ❏ Urimax
- ❏ Urised
- ❏ Urispas
- ❏ Uritin
- ❏ Urobiotic
- ❏ Urocit
- ❏ Uroquid
- ❏ Uroplus
- ❏ Urotrol
- ❏ UroXatral
- ❏ Vagistat
- ❏ Vancocin
- ❏ Vantin
- ❏ Vaprisol
- ❏ VESIcare
- ❏ Vibramycin
- ❏ Vibra-Tabs
- ❏ Vinarol
- ❏ Vincol
- ❏ Virilon
- ❏ Vivelle
- ❏ YM178
- ❏ Zinacef
- ❏ Zithromax
- ❏ Zithromax Z-Pak
- ❏ Zyloprim

VACCINES

- ❑ 13 Valent Vaccine
- ❑ ACAM2000
- ❑ Acel-Imune
- ❑ ActHIB
- ❑ Adacel
- ❑ Advate
- ❑ Afluria
- ❑ Agriflu
- ❑ Aidsvax
- ❑ Anthrax
- ❑ Attenuvax
- ❑ Bacillus Calmette-Guerin
- ❑ Bay-Gam
- ❑ Bay-Hep
- ❑ Bay-Rab
- ❑ Bay-Rho
- ❑ Bay-Tet
- ❑ BIAVAX
- ❑ BioThrax
- ❑ Boostrix
- ❑ Calmette-Guerin
- ❑ Certiva
- ❑ Cervarix
- ❑ Cholera
- ❑ Comvax
- ❑ CytoGam
- ❑ Daptacel
- ❑ Digibind
- ❑ diphtheria
- ❑ Dryvax
- ❑ DTP
- ❑ Engerix-B
- ❑ Fluarix
- ❑ FluLaval
- ❑ Fluogen
- ❑ FluShield
- ❑ Fluvirin
- ❑ Fluzone

VACCINES

- ❑ Gamimune
- ❑ Gammagard
- ❑ Gammar
- ❑ Gardasil
- ❑ H1N1
- ❑ H5N1
- ❑ haemophilus b
- ❑ Havrix
- ❑ H-Big
- ❑ HDCV
- ❑ hepatitis
- ❑ Hiberix
- ❑ Hibtiter
- ❑ HyperRab
- ❑ HyperTet
- ❑ HypRho-D
- ❑ Imogam
- ❑ Imovax
- ❑ Infanrix
- ❑ influenza
- ❑ Influenza A (H1N1)
- ❑ IPOL
- ❑ IPV
- ❑ Iveegam
- ❑ Ixiaro
- ❑ Je-Vax
- ❑ Kinrix
- ❑ LYMErix
- ❑ Measles
- ❑ Menactra
- ❑ MenACWY-CRM
- ❑ MenHibrix
- ❑ meningococcal conjugate
- ❑ Menomune
- ❑ Menveo
- ❑ Meruvax
- ❑ MICRhoGAM
- ❑ Movax

VACCINES

- ❑ M-M-R
- ❑ M-R Vax
- ❑ Mumpsvax
- ❑ Nab-HB
- ❑ OKA
- ❑ OmniHIB
- ❑ Optaflu
- ❑ OPV
- ❑ Orimune
- ❑ OspA
- ❑ PedvaxHIB
- ❑ Pentacel
- ❑ Pertussis
- ❑ pneumococcal 13-valent
- ❑ Pneumovax
- ❑ Pnu-Immune
- ❑ poliomyelitis
- ❑ Poliovax
- ❑ Prevnar
- ❑ Prevnar 13
- ❑ ProHIBiT
- ❑ Proquad
- ❑ Provenge
- ❑ RabAvert
- ❑ Recombinant QspA
- ❑ Recombivax HB
- ❑ RhoGAM
- ❑ Rickettsia
- ❑ Rotarix
- ❑ RotaShield
- ❑ rotavirus
- ❑ Rubella
- ❑ Rubeola
- ❑ Sabin
- ❑ Salk
- ❑ Sandoglobulin
- ❑ smallpox
- ❑ SparVax

VACCINES

- ❑ T.A.B.
- ❑ Takeda pertussis
- ❑ TE Anatoxal Berna
- ❑ Tetanus toxoid
- ❑ Tetramune
- ❑ Theracys
- ❑ TICE BCG
- ❑ TOPV
- ❑ TriHibit
- ❑ Tri-Immunol
- ❑ Tripedia
- ❑ tuberculosis
- ❑ Twinrix
- ❑ Typhim
- ❑ Typhoid
- ❑ vaccinia
- ❑ Vaqta
- ❑ varicella
- ❑ Varivax
- ❑ Vivotef Berna
- ❑ VZIG
- ❑ WinRho
- ❑ whooping cough
- ❑ YF-Vax
- ❑ Zemaira
- ❑ Zostavax
- ❑ zoster

X-RAY MEDIUMS

- ❑ 99mmTC
- ❑ 99mmTcDTPA
- ❑ Abrodil
- ❑ Acctiodonc
- ❑ Acetrizoate
- ❑ Acetrizoic acid
- ❑ Albumotrope

X-RAY MEDIUMS

- ❏ Aldosterone
- ❏ Amyvid
- ❏ AN-DTPA Kit
- ❏ Angio-Conray
- ❏ Angiopac
- ❏ Angiotensin
- ❏ Apcitide
- ❏ Areteray
- ❏ Arteriodone
- ❏ Baridol
- ❏ Bariform
- ❏ barium sulfate
- ❏ Barosperse
- ❏ Barotrast
- ❏ BAS 16
- ❏ Bilgrafin
- ❏ Biliodyl
- ❏ Bilitrast
- ❏ Bilopaque
- ❏ Biloptin
- ❏ Bilospect
- ❏ bismuth carbonate
- ❏ calcium ipodate
- ❏ Campiodol
- ❏ CardioGen 82
- ❏ Cardiografin
- ❏ CardioTec Kit
- ❏ Cardiotrast
- ❏ CEA-SCAN
- ❏ Cesium 137
- ❏ chloriodized oil
- ❏ cholebrine
- ❏ Cholepelvis
- ❏ Choleradiagnostic
- ❏ Cholestim
- ❏ Cholevic
- ❏ Cholografin
- ❏ chromalbin

X-RAY MEDIUMS

- ❏ chromic phosphate
- ❏ chromitope sodium
- ❏ Cis-Pyro Kit
- ❏ cobalt
- ❏ colloidal barium sulfate
- ❏ Conray
- ❏ cortisol
- ❏ Cysto-Conray
- ❏ deoxycorticosterone
- ❏ Diaginol
- ❏ Diagnorenol
- ❏ Diatrast
- ❏ diatrizoate
- ❏ digitoxin
- ❏ digoxin T-125
- ❏ Dimer-X
- ❏ Diodrast
- ❏ Dionosil
- ❏ diphosphonate
- ❏ disodium etidronate
- ❏ esriol
- ❏ Esophotrast
- ❏ ethiodized oil
- ❏ Ethiodol
- ❏ ferumoxide
- ❏ florbetapir F 18
- ❏ fluorescein
- ❏ Gadavist
- ❏ gadiodiamide
- ❏ gadobutrol
- ❏ gallium citrate
- ❏ Gastrografin
- ❏ GastroMark
- ❏ Glofil-125
- ❏ Gold AU 198
- ❏ HD-85
- ❏ Hexabrix
- ❏ Hippuran I 131

X-RAY MEDIUMS

- Hipputope
- hyaluronidase
- Hylenex
- Hypaque
- Hyskon
- Hytone
- Hytrast
- IC_Green
- Indium
- indocyanine green
- Iocetamic acid
- Iohexol
- iophendylate
- iothalamate
- ipodate
- Isopaque
- Lipiodol
- MDP kit
- meglumine
- methylglucamine
- metrizamide
- MMA kit
- MPI Iodine
- Myoview
- NeoTect
- Omnipaque
- Omniscan
- Oragrafin
- Oratrast
- OsteoScan
- Perchloracap
- pertechnetate sodium
- Phosphocol
- progesterone RIA
- propyliodone

X-RAY MEDIUMS

- Quantisorb
- Renografin
- Reno-M-30
- Renotec
- Renovist
- Rubratope
- Salpix
- selenomethionine
- Sensor
- Sinaografin
- sodium chromate
- sodium diatrizoate
- sodium diphosphate
- sodium iodide
- sodium iodohippurate
- sodium pertechnetate
- sodium phosphate
- sodium rose Bengal
- sodium tyropanoate
- Strontium
- Technescan
- Technetium
- Telepaque
- Tensilon
- Tetrasorb
- Thyrolute
- Thyrostat
- Thyrotropin Alfa
- tricarbocyanine
- triolein
- Triosorb
- Vascoray
- Visipaque
- XE 133
- Xenon